LABOUR OF

LABOUR OF LOVE

The Story of the World's First Surrogate Grandmother

SUE REID

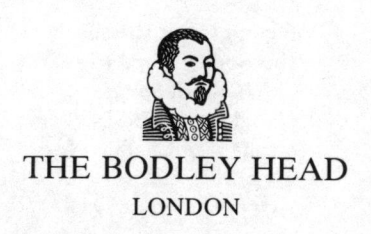

THE BODLEY HEAD
LONDON

Photographs 1 to 4 reproduced courtesy of the Anthony and Ferreira-Jorge families. Photographs 5 to 31 taken by Lynn Hilton and David O'Neill, copyright Mail Newspapers PLC.

Article by A.N. Wilson from the *Daily Mail* reproduced by kind permission of the *Daily Mail*.

A CIP catalogue record for this book is available from the British Library.

ISBN: 0–370–31236–8 (Pbk)

© Sue Reid/*Mail on Sunday* 1988

Printed in Great Britain for
The Bodley Head Ltd,
32 Bedford Square,
London WC1B 3EL
by Mackays of Chatham Ltd

First published in 1988

With thanks to the *Mail on Sunday* team:
Lynn Hilton, Adrian Lithgow, Peter Day,
Keith Waldegrave, Chester Stern, Chris Cousins,
David O'Neill and Graeme Gourlay

Acknowledgements

Life magazine, Time Inc., Chicago; *Baby Cotton: For Love and Money* by Kim Cotton and Denise Winn, Dorling Kindersley, London; *In Vitro Fertilisation Past, Present, Future* edited by S. Fishel and E.M. Symonds, IRL Press, Oxford; *Test-Tube Conception* by Professor Carl Wood and Ann Westmore, George Allen and Unwin, London

Contents

List of photographs	viii
Chapter 1	1
Chapter 2	12
Chapter 3	24
Chapter 4	37
Chapter 5	48
Chapter 6	60
Chapter 7	74
Chapter 8	87
Chapter 9	102
Chapter 10	113

List of Photographs

1. Pat Anthony with baby Karen.
2. Karen's wedding to Alcino Ferreira-Jorge. Left to right: Karen's brother Colin, Pat Anthony, Alcino, Karen, Raymond Anthony.
3. Karen with newly born Alcino Junior.
4. Karen and Alcino with Alcino Junior.
5 and 6. Pat Anthony and husband Raymond.
7. Karen and Alcino with Pat.
8. Karen and her mother in April 1987, three months into the pregnancy.
9. Pat with Karen and Alcino in April 1987.
10 and 11. Pat, Karen, Alcino and Alcino Junior during the pregnancy.
12 and 13. The Ferreira-Jorges with Pat at the Park Lane Clinic shortly before the birth.
14. Staff from the Vita Lab Clinic.
15, 16 and 17. (left to right) Drs Joel Bernstein and Cecil Michelow of the Vita Lab Clinic and Dr Johan Van Der Wat, Pat Anthony's original gynaecologist.
18. Baby Jose, the second of the triplets to arrive, is held up triumphantly in the delivery room.
19. Karen with the newly born triplets, David, Jose and Paula.

20. Karen, Alcino and Raymond in an emotional embrace outside the delivery room.
21. Karen and Alcino admire David, the first born of the triplets.
22. Alcino Junior meets one of the babies.
23 and 24. Raymond Anthony and his grandson Alcino Junior with the new members of their family.
25, 26 and 27. Pat and the Ferreira-Jorges getting to know the triplets during the first few days after the birth.
28. Following weeks of preparation, Karen is able to breast-feed her babies.
29. The unique family: grandmother Pat with Karen, Alcino and the triplets.
30 and 31. Seven months on: Karen, Alcino and Pat with Alcino Junior, David, Jose and Paula during a trip to England in May 1988.

Chapter 1

Karen Ferreira-Jorge had everything to live for on the night of her mother Pat's 45th-birthday party at the El Toro Steak House in her home town of Tzaneen, a thriving avocado-farming community in the fertile Letaba Valley of South Africa's Northern Transvaal. Not only did this vivacious 22-year-old relish the family reunion, but she was about to give birth to the baby she had always longed for.

On that hot evening of 23 February 1984, late in the southern hemisphere's summer, the dinner for eight family and friends was drawing to a close as the chatter turned to Karen's superbly healthy pregnancy and discussion about whether the imminent new arrival would be a boy or a girl.

All day Karen, who sipped grape juice throughout the party, had been having odd contractions signalling that the baby would soon be on the way. Since her marriage the year before she had been consumed with an ambition for motherhood and, like her 30-year-old Portuguese husband Alcino, she was very excited.

So too was Pat, her petite and good-natured mother, who that evening was careful to hide her disappointment that her first grandchild would not now share her birthdate. At the head of that happy table at the El Toro was Karen's 44-year-old father Raymond, a Tzaneen shop owner who, after a tumbler or two of his favourite imported Scotch whisky, announced to his family that he hoped for a grandson.

Through her 40 weeks of pregnancy Karen had thrived with the child growing inside her. She had declared most publicly to her female friends, and indeed anyone who cared to listen, that her ideal was to have a large family of four or five children. Babies, she said, were to be the most important part of her life and her marriage.

She had suffered from morning sickness right from the beginning, but stoically completed her weekly ante-natal exercise classes without any complaint. This mother-to-be had planned a textbook-perfect pregnancy and had read everything she could about birth and babies. She was determined that, although she was to have the child at the 40-bed Van Velden Memorial Hospital in Tzaneen, it would be a natural birth.

Like many of the white English-speaking girls she had grown up with at her state-run weekly boarding school, The Capricorn High in Pietersburg, 90 kilometres away from Tzaneen, Karen had never sought out a career. She had been raised protectively in the bosom of a Lebanese family where being a good mother and caring wife still rated far more highly than independence and earning a pay packet.

If Karen's hopes seemed simple, even old-fashioned, it was because she had been kept sheltered in the small town near the Mozambique border through all her 22 years. If she was innocent, it was because her strict parents had watched over their only daughter, never letting her out too late in the evenings, always being there to pick her up in the family's white Mercedes from the local parties, and vetting closely her visits to the films showing at the open-air cinema, the quaintly named Bioscope. When she left school at 16 Karen worked in a Tzaneen dress shop and lived at home, never seeking out the bright lights of Johannesburg. And even at 22 she was not allowed to drive through her home town alone.

At the end of that memorable birthday party Karen

kissed her mother goodnight. The two were close and telephoned each other every day, although Karen had been married for almost a year. Then she was carefully driven home by Alcino, through the tropical Tzaneen night, to the modest rented flat near the town's centre where the two had made their first home.

It was during the small hours that her pains started and the next morning Karen left the flat with her neatly packed overnight case. At 7.30 she was delivered by Alcino in their Ford Escort to the main entrance of the Van Velden Hospital, just four minutes' drive away.

No one could possibly have suspected what was to come. No one could ever have predicted that within 24 hours of Karen kissing her husband goodbye in the hospital lobby, she would lie dying with her new baby son crying alone in the nursery nearby.

'Alcino went to work that morning and told his boss he wouldn't be staying for long because I had gone into labour. All day everything went very well and by 10 in the evening I was in the second stage of labour,' says Karen.

With Alcino with her, holding her hand in the delivery room, Alcino Junior was born at 11.50 p.m. on 24 February. The delighted couple had already decided on the name if their child was a boy. 'It had all been the most wonderful experience of my life and I will never forget it.'

The new mother held the baby in her arms for five minutes after the birth, then he was lifted away to be washed. The doctor and nurses asked Karen to push once again to get rid of the afterbirth or placenta. She tried and tried but nothing at all happened. Very soon the medical team realized that something was going horribly wrong. Suddenly the perfect pregnancy was over.

Standing by Karen's side was the local doctor, tall but gentle Louis Boezaart, a friend of Raymond and Pat Anthony who had known her since she was a girl. After a few minutes he grew alarmed that the stubborn placenta had still not arrived. Finally he leant over the young mother and told her quietly that he would have to take her into the operating theatre and remove the after birth by hand. His words were the last that Karen would remember or understand for many hours.

In the small theatre, the unconscious Karen's placenta was finally removed and Dr Boezaart watched as she was wheeled back to the white-walled maternity ward of the hospital. He believed that all would be well. He sent Alcino, who sat waiting in the hospital corridor, out into the night to celebrate his fatherhood with his parents-in-law at their penthouse flat above their haberdashery and gift shop in the high street of Tzaneen. And then the doctor checked the mother and baby one more time before going home himself.

But half an hour later Karen still lay unconscious, and a nursing sister passing her bedside noticed that blood was seeping through the narrow mattress beneath her body on to the lino floor below. When the sister checked Karen's pulse there seemed to be absolutely none. She ran to the telephone to ring Dr Boezaart's home and told the stunned doctor that the Ferreira-Jorge girl looked as though she was already dead.

'There had been absolutely no problems with the delivery of Alcino Junior,' says Boezaart. 'The birth was just about as uncomplicated as it could be. What happened next was like a bomb that exploded without the slightest warning.'

In a few minutes Dr Boezaart had driven back to the hospital from his house nearby and was fighting to bring Karen back to life. He shouted at her, carried out frantic heart massage and mouth-to-mouth resuscitation. Very slowly her pulse returned.

At just before one o'clock in the morning, the telephone rang at Raymond and Pat's flat, as Alcino sipped champagne and told his parents-in-law about the excitement of the birth. It was Dr Boezaart on the other end of the line, and he instructed Alcino to drive immediately across the Transvaal to Duiwelskloof to the nearest blood-bank and 'bring as much O-negative blood as it holds'. With

Raymond he set off, completing what was usually a 40-minute return journey in half that time.

The two arrived back at Ven Velden Hospital to find that Karen's 21-year-old brother, Colin, had already been called to donate blood as had the matron in charge. 'As they gave me the blood it was just coming out of me again,' says Karen. 'They even called in all the local blood donors. One man stood next to me as they transfused his blood straight into my bloodstream.'

Alcino was deeply shocked. He was already in tears outside Karen's ward when he overheard a hospital administrator making an emergency call to Dr Paul Duminy, a gynaecologist from Pietersburg Hospital. 'Come quickly,' said the administrator to Duminy. 'But I don't think she'll still be alive when you get here.'

During that long night Karen was revived three times and 17 pints of blood were poured into her body. By the time Dr Duminy arrived with a police escort there were fears that she had irreparable brain damage because her pupils had dilated.

Duminy and Boezaart decided that Karen must have an immediate hysterectomy. 'The placenta had grown into my uterus instead of just attaching to it,' explains Karen. 'When Dr Boezaart decided to remove my placenta manually he had pulled it and, of course, I bled. I also had an embolism, because the fluid from my uterus entered my bloodstream, stopping my blood clotting properly.'

The doctors believed that if Karen survived at all it would be as a vegetable. But as dawn broke over Tzaneen they went ahead with the operation. It would, they knew, mean the end of childbearing for this 22-year-old, yet there was simply no choice if her life was to be saved. At 5.30 a distraught Alcino was asked to sign the medical forms giving his permission for the hysterectomy and once again Karen was wheeled into the hospital's little theatre and put under anaesthetic.

As soon as her uterus was removed Karen's pupils stopped dilating, her pulse returned to normal and the bleeding which had drained her body stopped. And at breakfast time she was driven by ambulance to the intensive care unit of Pietersburg Hospital, with the baby in a cot by her side.

All Karen could recall when she woke for the first time in the ambulance was that she had given birth to a baby boy the night before. Then she went back to sleep, mercifully still unaware of how nearly she had died or that she would never again enjoy a pregnancy.

For the next 24 hours Karen slipped in and out of consciousness and breathed with the help of tubes in the intensive care unit. She was so ill that she never questioned why she was in a strange place and without the baby. On the Saturday afternoon three 'get-well' telegrams arrived from friends in Tzaneen. 'The nursing sister made a mistake and read them to me,' says Karen. 'The hospital wanted them kept quiet in case I realized I was so ill. But even when I had heard them I didn't put two and two together and think that something was wrong. I just kept going back to sleep.'

On the Sunday of that gruelling weekend Karen, with Alcino Junior nearly two days old, was told the truth that would shatter her happiness. The previous day Alcino had visited Karen and prepared to break the news of the hysterectomy but his young wife looked so weak he did not have the courage.

Instead it was left to Dr Duminy to have one of the most difficult conversations of his medical career. Soon after Karen was wheeled from the intensive care unit to the maternity ward, he told the woman who wanted to dedicate her life to her babies that there could never be any more children for her. She was thoroughly in love with her husband too and wanted to please him by providing a large and healthy family. She now had one baby, but would that ever be enough to satisfy her strong maternal cravings?

'Things went wrong at the birth, you lost a lot of blood and we have had to remove your uterus to save your life,' Duminy told Karen. 'You have had a total hysterectomy.'

Karen knew exactly what that operation entailed and deep inside she realized what the future held but still she persisted vainly in asking, 'And what does that mean to me?' Dr Duminy leaned forward towards her, trying to make the harsh words seem less forbidding, 'It means you will never be able to have children again'.

Karen didn't burst into tears. The news hardly sank in at that point because she was so exhausted, too muddled by the events of the last 48 hours for the real cruelty of her situation to become clear. Indeed she was so ill that she was near to rejecting her own baby.

The nurse kept coming to me and asking if she could bring up my new child from the hospital nursery, but I just said no. I was so tired and disappointed with everything that I didn't even want to start thinking about looking after a baby.

That afternoon her parents and husband visited her, and it was then that Karen's emotions showed themselves for the first time. At the sight of Alcino, Raymond and Pat, she broke down completely. And when the baby was carried in a few minutes later she admits, 'It was the first realization for me of what had really happened. I was a mother, I had given birth, but I would never ever be able to do so again.'

Her mother, father and Alcino clustered around the crib and talked, like families do, about who the baby looked like. 'I was only able to lie there and watch. I was so drawn that my mother had to feed me soup with a spoon. I couldn't even find the strength to pick up the bowl.'

Pat had remained calm throughout the family's ordeal. On the night Alcino Junior was born she went to Tzaneen hospital and prayed silently outside Karen's room. And even though her only daughter was seriously ill she walked along to the hospital nursery to check that her grandchild, lying in an incubator, was bathed and not hungry.

'I was grateful to the doctors for saving Karen's life. I had prayed she would not be taken from us or her baby of only a few hours old,' she recalled, quietly and philosophically. Though a devout Roman Catholic, Pat has never been a woman to flaunt her beliefs. To her prayer is a very personal thing between man and God.

> When the doctors decided to do the hysterectomy and Alcino signed the forms, I knew immediately what it would do to Karen. She wanted more children, she had enjoyed every single day of her pregnancy, and even the birth itself. I dreaded her waking up to find out she was barren. But it was the only way to save her.

For Alcino too this was a harrowing time. Every night without fail he would visit Karen, grey with his sadness and disappointment that the birth of his first child had turned out so tragically. But he was outwardly strong for Karen's sake. To him fatherhood stood for everything. As a 21-year-old, nine years before, he had left his own country, Portuguese-run Angola, as it slid towards Marxism at the end of colonial rule. He had been raised in a self-made family which had prospered from farming and trading in a land where labour was cheap and plentiful.

Leaving his mother crying on the porch, Alcino had fled his family's eight-bedroomed house in Nova Lisboa, and set off on a remarkable three-day journey towards a fresh life in South Africa. He had no passport or papers with him, so he could not be identified if stopped by the rebel troops. And he came across the border into south-west Africa carrying only a box of hand grenades, a small suitcase and two loaded rifles.

Without an English word between them, Alcino, with his elder brother Almiro, sister-in-law Dina and the couple's baby son, made the flight to South Africa in a battered beige Opel car. At times the brothers pushed the old car through the bush with the engine turned off so that they would not be heard. They avoided proper roads and searched for safe routes towards the border. When they finally arrived in south-west Africa on a dirt track they had no inkling of exactly where they were on the map.

Yet to their amazement the soldiers who surrounded the car as it skidded to a halt were South African troops who were patrolling the border and the Portuguese family were welcomed. After less than a month in one of the state refugee camps, first in South Africa's political capital, Pretoria, and then in Johannesburg, Alcino was offered a job in a town he had never even heard of. The job was as a refrigeration engineer. The town was Tzaneen.

It was a lonely time for Alcino, isolated because he could not speak or write either English or Afrikaans. By day he would work at Jackamans, the Tzaneen refrigeration engineering firm, and by evening he acted as an usher at the Bioscope. It was a way of meeting people and practising his new languages.

And it was at the Bioscope that he was to be introduced to Karen, just a few months after his arrival as a refugee. 'At first I thought she was much too young for me, after all, she was still a schoolgirl. But I could see she liked me too. I didn't stop trying to take her out.' He smiles.

But Raymond and Pat Anthony were not enamoured with the idea of their 15-year-old daughter becoming seriously involved with a man six years her senior who did not speak English. They had always hoped their only daughter would marry into the close-knit Lebanese community from which they had come. Raymond fought against the blossoming relationship between the schoolgirl and the refugee. He argued, with the backing of the more patient Pat, that it was too early for Karen to be seeing one boyfriend regularly and there were a number of serious family rows. Finally the hot-tempered Raymond ordered the couple to stop meeting for a year.

Karen had never had a boyfriend before and once she met Alcino she was never to have another. It was a love match which, despite the strong parental opposition and enforced separations, ended happily enough with their marriage at the local Roman Catholic church in Tzaneen on 1 May 1983 when Karen was still only 21.

'We always said that when we were married we wanted children, as many as possible. We agreed that we'd have to start straight away to get that right. After the first month, when I didn't fall pregnant, Alcino was very upset. And then suddenly during the second month I had a secret to tell him . . .'

It was a joyous moment for the girl who had always longed for babies. She immediately went down to the shops in Tzaneen, bought a pair of yellow booties and wrapped them up. Then she drove to the front gate of Jackamans, on the outskirts of the town, and waited for Alcino to come out of work at five in the evening.

'He opened up the parcel of booties and I had written a card telling him we were going to have a baby. He just went very quiet but we were both very happy that day,' recalls Karen.

Before their marriage Alcino and Karen had talked about what would happen if they were not blessed with children. They had even discussed the merits of adoption, but Alcino had insisted from the start that he would not be able to accept such a thing. Although after the tragic events following Alcino Junior's birth he was to tell his grieving wife he had changed his mind about adopting a baby, it was an option they never took really seriously. 'It made me feel a lot better to know we could do this if it came to the crunch,' remembers Karen. 'But we never even put our names down on a list or anything.'

However, as Karen recovered slowly at Pietersburg Hospital, learning for the first time to breast-feed a baby, a remarkable thing happened. She did not realize its significance then and it would take two more years for its importance to become apparent.

Just four days after Karen nearly died, Alcino went to the Pietersburg Hospital with a message from his sister-in-law Dina, who had shared the Portuguese family's dramatic flight to South Africa from Angola nearly a decade earlier.

Dina, he told Karen, had offered to become a surrogate mother for her. She would be prepared to carry their baby and then hand it over to them when it was born. Although Dina lived far away in Sasolberg in the Free State, she had sent this message to Karen. It was a great gesture of love and sympathy from a woman who was not a blood relative and already had two boys of her own to look after.

Says Karen:

I had never even heard of the word surrogate then and I had no idea that a woman could carry another woman's child. I responded to Alcino by exclaiming that it was a good idea, but I really didn't know what to say. It was only later, when I was alone, that I started to think about it earnestly. As the weeks went by it was more and more on my mind.

This was the moment when the first seeds of the idea that surrogacy might be a possible solution were sown. As yet the new baby was still a stranger to Karen and for the time being she was preoccupied with caring for him, and getting to know his little foibles, strengths and weaknesses. But as time went on the idea was to become more firmly lodged in her mind.

Meanwhile, in Britain, the first commercial surrogacy, which led to the birth in January 1985 of Baby Cotton in a North London hospital, was still being covertly planned. Twenty-eight-year-old Kim Cotton, the British housewife who carried Baby Cotton for a payment of £6,500, did not become pregnant until 13 April 1984, six weeks after Karen and Alcino's momentous conversation at the hospital's visiting time. Yet this idea of surrogacy, which was relatively unknown in Britain, let alone in an obscure South African town, was something that Karen Ferreira-Jorge was never to forget.

Chapter 2

It was a very resolute Pat Anthony who arrived at the consulting rooms of her gynaecologist, Dr Johan Van Der Wat, at 12.15 on Tuesday 10 June 1986. Although this diminutive woman of four foot 11 inches was not known for spirited independence, her heritage was Lebanese and in such households a grandmother's word is often revered. That day she had an important question to put to the doctor and if it was answered to her satisfaction it would alter the path of her daughter's life and her own.

Pat had been staying for a week in Johannesburg with close friends, Mandy and Cliffie Jacob, at their unpretentious but welcoming family house at the end of a quiet cul-de-sac called Berry Avenue. It was in this house, in the city's southern suburb of Oakdene, that Pat would later hide away from the world, and in particular the South African press, during her pregnancy.

On this Tuesday, just approaching the South African winter, it was all arranged that she would be returning to Tzaneen at midday. She was to be picked up from Berry Avenue by her 22-year-old son, Colin, who was on his way home in the family Mercedes from Grahamstown University in the Cape to the Northern Transvaal for his student vacation.

Yet in the middle of the morning Pat suddenly altered the long-standing arrangement with her son. Colin, she instructed, was now to collect her at 12.45, not from the Berry Avenue house but from the Park Lane Clinic, Johannesburg. Then she swiftly and secretly picked up the telephone in Mandy's dining room and called Dr Van Der Wat's receptionist to say she must see the doctor urgently.

The faithful Mandy, a hairdresser with a salon in Oakdene, drove her friend to the hospital, a 20-minute ride away into the city on Johannesburg's M1. Pat did not tell Mandy the purpose of her visit to the doctor's, only that Dr Van Der Wat had some test results ready for her, following a quite genuine consultation some weeks before about whether she had reached the menopause.

As she entered the lift of the busy clinic and rode up to the first floor to look for room 2–11, she was delighted the doctor had agreed to see her so promptly. It did not give her time to lose her courage or to hesitate about posing the vital question.

Van Der Wat had no inkling of what the 47-year-old grandmother from Tzaneen wanted. And it was only when Pat was perched in the red leather armchair in front of his solid oak desk that he realized it was no ordinary consultation. On the previous visit Pat had told him that her 24-year-old daughter, Karen, was married with a two-year-old son. She had confided that Karen was deeply depressed following the hysterectomy which had been performed after the birth of Alcino Junior. Her daughter was desperate to have more children but that, Pat had explained to the sympathetic Van Der Wat, was impossible.

Now Pat prepared herself to make a momentous personal plea to the gynaecologist, himself a father of four children under ten years old. Pat asked if she could become a surrogate mother for Karen. Could she carry her own grandchild? Was she young enough, fit enough and anyway, was it a medical possibility?

Van Der Wat, a dedicated doctor who often used to say, in all seriousness but with a twinkle in his eye, 'I will do anything to help women make babies,' listened intently as she talked. Pat explained that on Karen's 24th birthday a few weeks before a young friend had noticed that her daughter was visibly depressed. At the birthday party in Tzaneen the friend, Jill Hoetz, had approached Karen and offered to be a surrogate mother for her.

Surrogacy was thankfully not a new concept to Dr Van Der Wat, nor was he hostile then, or now, to the idea of one woman carrying another's baby, especially if it was all kept in the family. Unlike many South African doctors he never used the Republic's isolation from the rest of the world as an excuse for not keeping abreast of new medical breakthroughs.

As a prominent Afrikaner and senior figure in the Dutch Reformed Church, which is hostile to surrogacy, this doctor could have put an end to Pat's extraordinary plan there and then. But instead, he was broad-minded enough to sweep away the doubts and tell Pat that he was willing to help her in any way he could.

Van Der Wat said:

Pat was very positive about becoming a surrogate. From tests I had done on her earlier I knew that it was possible for her to carry her daughter's child although she was 47. In fact, I told her there were a lot of things in her favour. Her health was still good, her change of life, although imminent, had not yet started, and she was obviously devoted to her daughter.

Although inwardly Van Der Wat was excited about the prospect of Pat bringing her daughter's baby into the world he was wary too. 'I told her exactly what could be done but insisted there was no absolute guarantee it would work. I said it was all brand new, this business of surrogacy, certainly when using a grandmother as the surrogate mother for her daughter's child.'

But Pat just listened eagerly as Van Der Wat, speaking incisively in his third language, English, told her to go home and discuss the whole idea with her family 300 miles away in Tzaneen. What he did not tell her was that if this

Mrs Anthony, a shopkeeper's wife from a small town in the Northern Transvaal, went ahead with her remarkable gesture of love, she would be a test case.

I had never read or heard of another grandmother wishing to carry her own grandchild. When Pat came to see me I had no knowledge of a 'gestational' surrogacy, where a woman is the incubator for the 'whole' embryo of another couple, happening anywhere else in the world. I thought it might have happened in Australia but I just didn't know. I believed we were probably on the brink of a world first. Anyway, in South Africa it was certainly a first. There had never been a surrogacy of any kind at all.

It had been an extraordinary discussion between this Roman Catholic grandmother and an Afrikaans doctor, but when Pat walked out of the Park Lane Clinic that day to the waiting Mercedes and her son Colin, she was sure there was no looking back.

In that vital half-hour of her secret visit, she had satisfied herself that there was no medical barrier to her carrying Karen and Alcino's baby. Against the very real odds in South Africa, she had opened her heart to a gynaecologist who was prepared to be positive.

As Pat travelled home that afternoon, she had time to think. There was no doubt that since Karen had become barren her whole disposition had changed. From being lively and outgoing she was now withdrawn and appeared deeply unhappy. The family had talked long and often about finding a surrogate, and Karen had even suggested searching overseas for a woman to carry her child.

'As Alcino Junior changed from baby into little boy, Karen seemed to get even more depressed,' recalls Pat. 'I wanted her to find a surrogate, I was not against the idea because I thought it would be nice for her. But ideally I thought it should be one of her close family, not a friend or a complete outsider.'

It was at seven that evening, when Pat was walking up the staircase to the Tzaneen penthouse, that she broke the astounding news of her decision to Karen. Karen remembers the moment well.

> I thought my mother had just been to Johannesburg for a general check-up, really just an excuse to get to Johannesburg, to go shopping and see her friends.
> Then I bumped into her as I came out of my father's penthouse and she told me that she had something important to say later. I wasn't having any of that, and I said if it is really important you must tell me now. And there we stood on the staircase while my mother explained how, secretly, she had seen her gynaecologist and he had said it was fine for her to carry our child. I was quite stunned. I didn't know what to say.

Even then Pat made two conditions about going ahead with the surrogacy.

> The first was that no one should ever know the identity of the surrogate mother. I wanted to remain absolutely anonymous, both in Tzaneen and everywhere else.
> I didn't want anyone to know it was me, and if necessary, I said we should pretend that Karen had been to Alcino's home country of Portugal and found a woman to do it. The second condition was that I would give up smoking, because I was getting through 60 a day then. I knew this worried Karen and I didn't want cigarettes to stand in the way of what I wanted to do for her.

Karen was anxious to tell Alcino, before anyone else was confided in. Her husband immediately pronounced the idea wonderful. He had always been close to Pat, even at the time when the family felt that his relationship with Karen was too serious. The Portuguese who had left his own parents in Angola 13 years before was on the same wave-length as Pat Anthony. They shared the same sense of humour, utterly confounding the antagonistic stereotype of mother-in-law and son-in-law.

But while Alcino, back at the three-bedroomed house on the outskirts of Tzaneen which he now rented with Karen, told his wife how wonderful it all was, underneath he was a worried man. 'Quite honestly, I was shocked. I was very thankful to Pat and I had no words to thank her then or now. But I never really believed it could possibly happen, mainly because of her age.'

At no time had the family ever considered Pat as a possible surrogate for Karen. But, after Alcino Junior's birth, 'whole' surrogacy had in theory become a realistic option for Karen. Every time she visited Dr Duminy for an annual check up at the Pietersburg Hospital, the first question on her lips was, 'Are my ovaries still working?' The answer was always yes and Karen would then ask another question. 'So, would it be possible to put my egg fertilized by Alcino's sperm into a surrogate mother?' The answer again was 'Yes'.

It is truly remarkable that a doctor in an isolated South African town, and a young woman who had hardly travelled outside the Republic could, in 1985, take such a possibility seriously. At that time there had been no 'host womb' surrogacies where the egg and sperm of one couple are placed in another woman for her to carry the embryo to birth. All successful surrogacies across Europe, in Australia and even in procreation-pioneering America had involved using the egg of the surrogate mother, with the only direct biological input of the childless couple being the husband's sperm.

In the United States Dr Wulf H. Utian, of the Mount Sinai Medical Centre in Cleveland, Ohio, was moving towards achieving a 'host-womb surrogacy', as these are now called. In 1984, a 42-year-old New York cardiologist and his wife, then aged 39, had approached this specialist in test-tube fertilization and asked, 'Why couldn't we get my wife's eggs, fertilize them with my sperm and have another woman to do the carrying?' Utian responded, 'But there's never been a case like this'.

It was only after meeting the couple, who remain anonymous, and discussing the ethical issues with his team alongside several religious leaders, that Dr Utian was persuaded to go ahead. But the first surrogate mother dropped out after three transfers failed and the difficulties served to underline how small the chances were of this kind of surrogacy working then and how problematic they still are now.

Meanwhile, in Britain, the test-tube pioneers the late Patrick Steptoe and Robert Edwards announced as recently as March 1986 that they wanted to start using a wife's eggs and husband's sperm to implant an embryo in a 'host' surrogate. Eight years earlier, in 1978, they were the two doctors who masterminded the birth of the world's first test-tube baby Louise Brown, at their laboratories in Oldham, Lancashire.

In the spring of 1986 Steptoe appealed to the British government, which by then had outlawed commercial surrogacy, to lay down guidelines for medically approved surrogacy, including the host womb or 'ghost parenting' method. But at the time Pamela Taylor, a spokeswoman for the British Medical Assocation, the watchdog body on ethics, declared crisply, 'This is an entirely new aspect of the controversy'. She added, 'We have no specific policy on this type of surrogacy'.

Yet across the world, in South Africa, Karen Ferreira-Jorge was determined to proceed, although it is clear that she was completely unaware of what uncharted waters she was steering into. By then she was reading avidly any magazine articles about surrogacy, but not even learned medical journals would have mentioned successful host womb births because none had happened at that time. However she insisted from the very start that if she and Alcino were to enlist the help of a surrogate mother, then she would have to carry their 'whole' biological baby.

She explains:

From the time I got home after Alcino Junior's birth I realized he might be the only one unless I did something about it. When I was left alone to simply get on with my life I found I was getting over-protective about the baby.

If the baby so much as coughed in the middle of the night, Alcino and Karen would fly out of bed to see what was wrong with him. Karen insisted that Alcino Junior should sleep right next to her in a cradle on the floor. At one stage she was getting up 17 times a night to make sure that he was still breathing. 'It was hitting me hard that I wasn't going to have any more children.'

She would weep to her husband, the bitter tears of a young woman who felt that she was being deprived.

I'd never cry to anybody else but Alcino was very understanding and patient. I found that for the first six or seven months I almost coped, but then when Alcino Junior was about ten months it became very bad. He was suddenly growing up, he started walking, and that was a big thing in our lives then.

But all I felt was that I was suddenly losing a baby, he was becoming a little boy so soon and I would never have the chance to have another little one. I had enjoyed him so much as a baby, you know.

It was when Alcino Junior was two that her father approached Karen and broached the idea of adoption. A straight-talking man, with little patience for fools, he insisted, 'If you want to adopt another baby you must at least put your names down. It doesn't just happen overnight.' The response from the strong-minded Karen was a cool rebuff, for she was already adamant that surrogacy was the answer.

'She had read about surrogacy happening overseas and believed that if she could still produce eggs then Alcino and she could have their own babies using a surrogate,' explains Raymond. 'Having their own biological child was the ultimate and Karen seemed prepared to wait until the technology caught up with her ideals.'

By the early days of 1986 Karen had received two offers from women willing to act as her surrogate. The first was from her sister-in-law, Dina, on that evening soon after Alcino Junior's birth when she had never even heard the word surrogate. Dina never went ahead with the idea because at the time she was living in the Free State, miles away from Tzaneen and from the doctors who would ultimately help Karen with her ambitious plan.

The second offer, which Pat had mentioned to Dr Van Der Wat, had come on Karen's 24th birthday. Karen remembers it well:

> We had a little party and a friend Jill Hoetz came to me and said she wanted to carry my baby for me. I was so shocked I didn't know what to say to her. At that stage we had started thinking about it and everyone knew we would really like to do it. But we didn't know where to go or where we were going to find a person to do it. Do we choose a person that we know, or do we choose a person that we don't know? Alcino and I had endless discussions.

On the night of the party Jill insisted she was serious about her offer, but Karen asked her what her husband thought of the idea. 'Later we spoke again and apparently her husband wasn't all for it because he understood, wrongly, that if she carried the babies they would be half her own. He didn't understand that the baby would be entirely Alcino's and mine.'

People ask Karen now whether she ever thought of turning to her mother and asking straight out for her to be the surrogate. She says no. 'I never actually believed she would be able to do it because of her age. I suppose I realized she was the one person who would be perfect, but not at 47 and with the change of life about to happen.'

Pat had met her husband Raymond more than 30 years

before when they were 12 years old, sitting in the Standard Five class of their secondary school in a South Johannesburg suburb, near Oakdene. The two Lebanese youngsters had taken no notice of each other, and a year later Raymond's family had moved away to Pretoria. It was only when he was a young man and returned to work on his father's market stall in Johannesburg that the two were to meet again and become close. Pat was working at that time in the office of a garage. Raymond remembers travelling home one night on the bus and spying Pat, whom he immediately sat next to.

'She was most reluctant to talk to me or go out with me. In fact —' he smiles ruefully '— she wasn't very keen at all. But I knew her mother well, being part of the same Lebanese community in Johannesburg and I got her mother on my side to arrange the first date. From there we just went along.'

It is a marriage that has stood up to the test of the years, through some hard times when money in the Anthony family was short and Pat, although by then the mother of two young children, helped supplement their income by doing bookkeeping and hairdressing. Their children were a comfort to them, and a joy. 'When they were born it was like nothing else that had ever happened in our lives,' says Raymond emotionally. 'It was like God's ultimate gift to us, and it made up for any difficulties.'

But following a very traumatic birth with Colin twenty-three years ago Pat had insisted to Raymond that she did not want any more children. By then they had moved to Tzaneen and started their shop. It was the perfect place, unlike the city, for a large and happy family to be reared. 'But I couldn't face going through another birth like that,' says Pat today. 'Two babies were enough for me. I was so lacking in calcium after having Karen and then Colin that my hair went very thin and I lost my teeth.'

That determination never to have another baby when Pat was 25 – the same age at which Karen was craving for more – might seem unremarkable now. But Pat and

Raymond came from families where traditionally four, five or six children would not be considered unusual. And that decision, nearly a quarter of a century ago, made her offer to carry Karen's child as a surrogate even more astonishing.

Raymond explained:

When Pat went off to see her gynaecologist in Johannesburg she actually cheated on me. She told me she was visiting Mandy and Cliffie Jacob and going to see the doctor there about having a hysterectomy. I tried to persuade her not to go. I said why don't you pay an initial visit to one of our local doctors and see what he says first of all. But she was so insistent that I just put it down to one of those women's things. I decided to play along with her even though, I admit now, I was getting a bit uptight about her having to leave the shop business and all the unnecessary travelling.

So when Pat returned from Johannesburg no one was more incredulous at her news than her own husband.

I was sitting reading in the drawing room of the penthouse when she just walked in and simply announced that with all the talking in the family about surrogacy she had done something about it. She told me she had been to Dr Van Der Wat in Johannesburg and been thoroughly checked, 100 per cent in every way that could be checked, and she was going to be the surrogate mother for Karen and Alcino's child.

Raymond admits now that he was devastated. 'I myself just clammed up because I never expected anything like this from my own wife. I thought it was a little bit of imagination although I supported the idea all along; there were initial fears too that her health would never stand up to it all.'

If Raymond, although he understood his wife well,

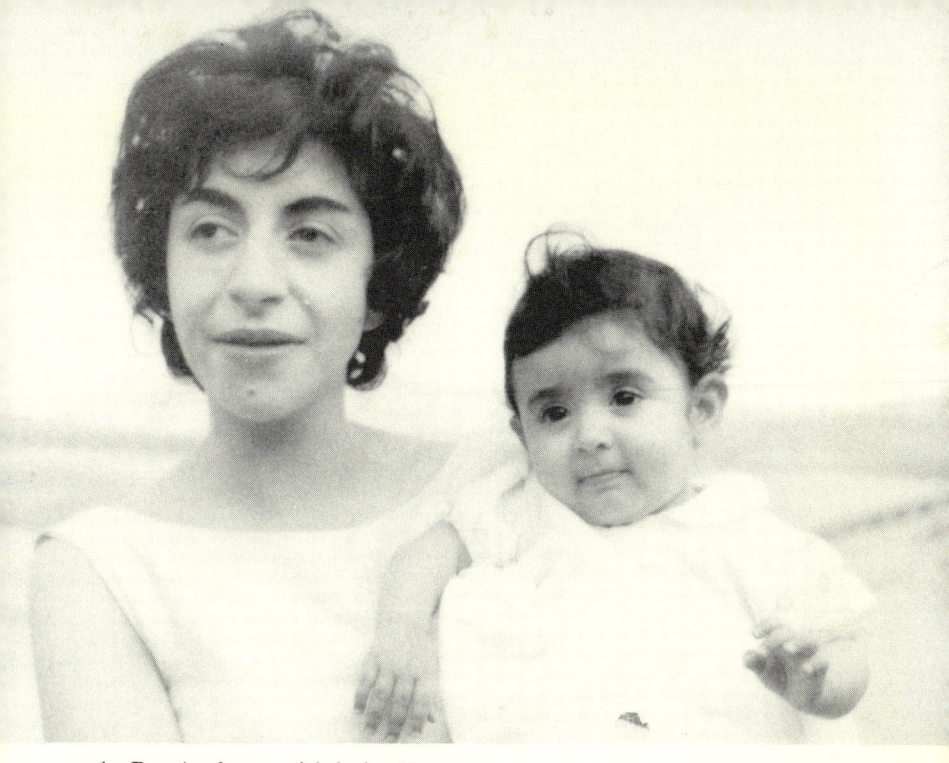

1. Pat Anthony with baby Karen.
2. Karen's wedding to Alcino Ferreira-Jorge. Left to right: Karen's brother Colin, Pat Anthony, Alcino, Karen, Raymond Anthony.

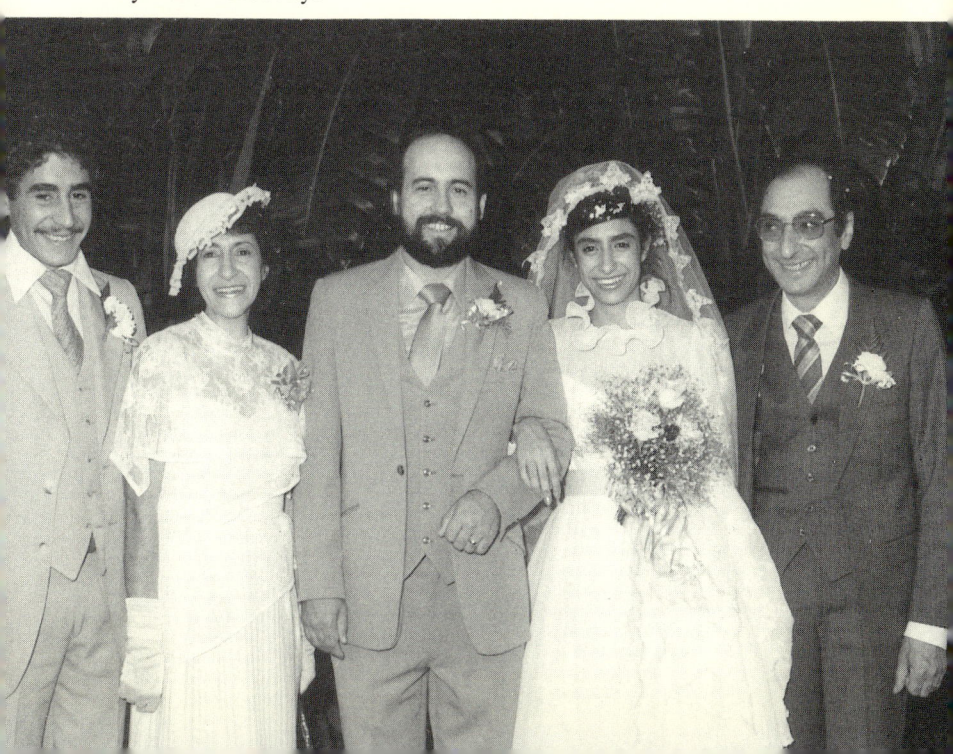

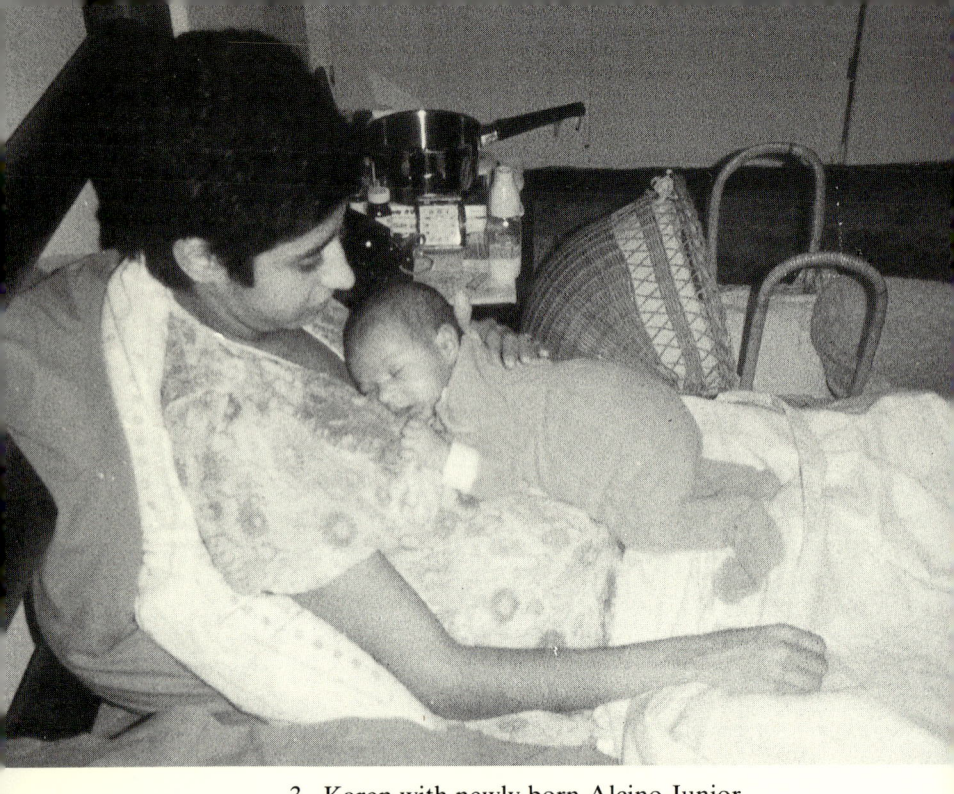

3. Karen with newly born Alcino Junior.
4. Karen and Alcino with Alcino Junior.

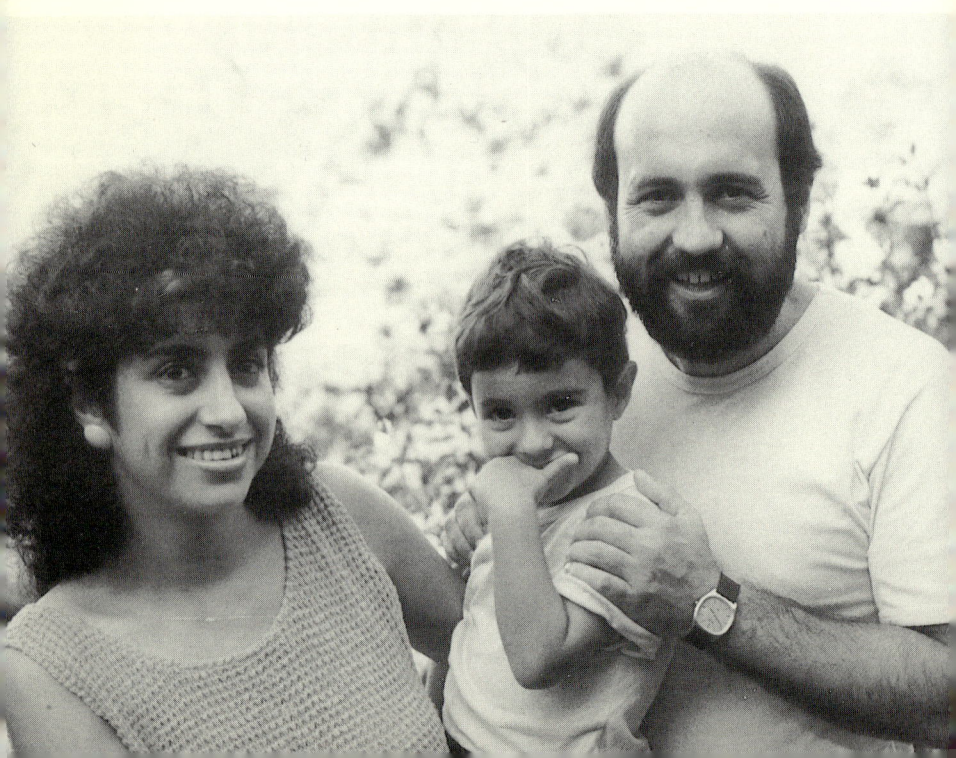

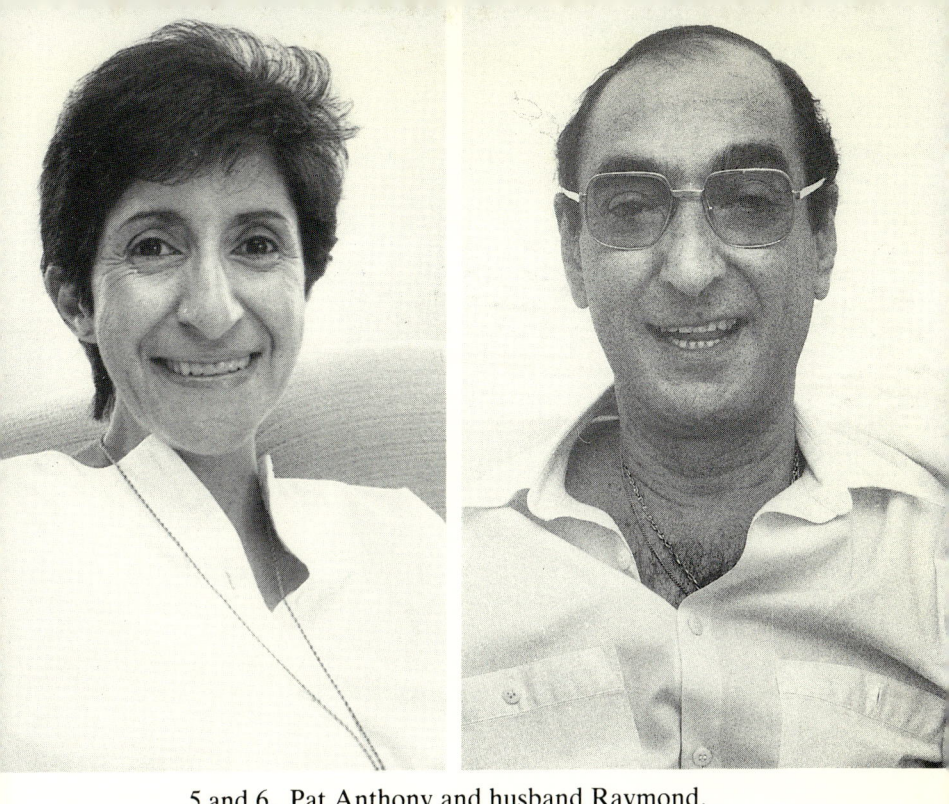

5 and 6. Pat Anthony and husband Raymond.
7. Karen and Alcino with Pat.

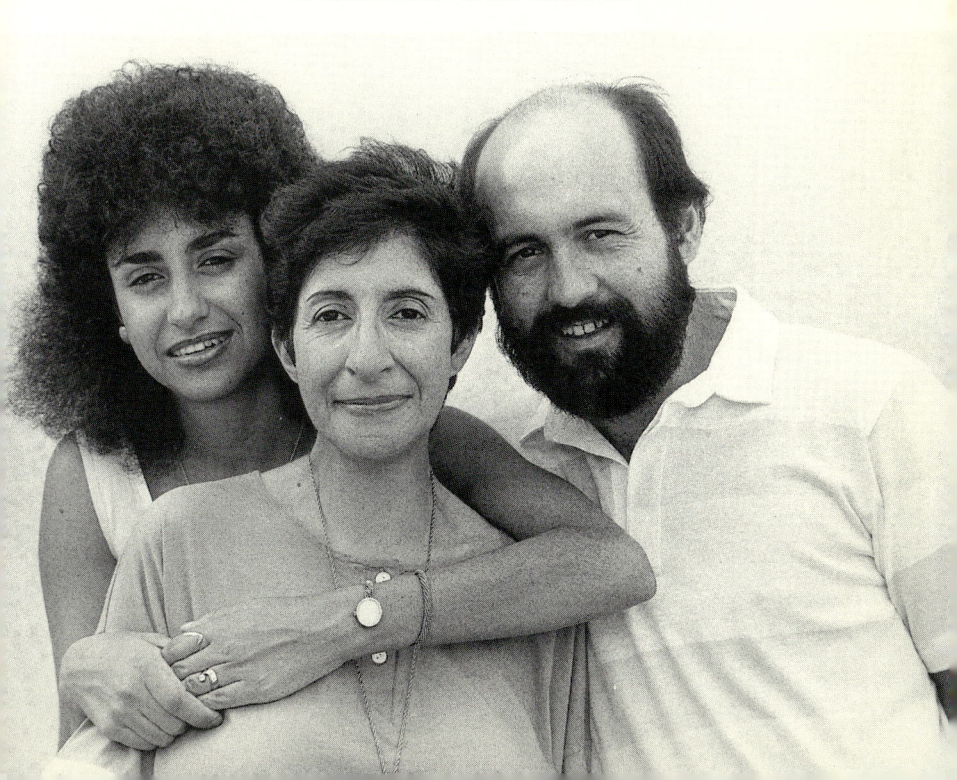

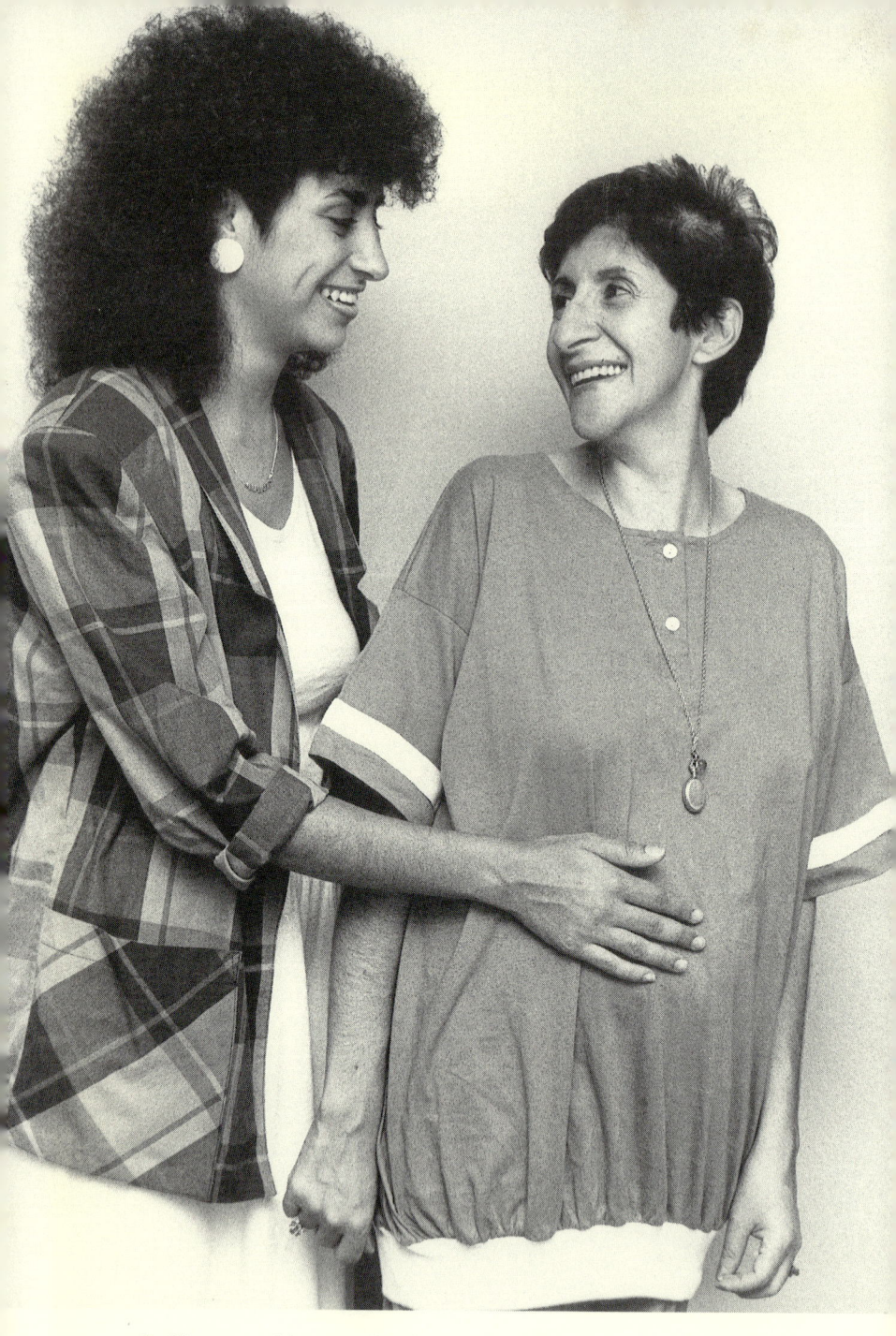

8. Karen and her mother in April, 1987, three months into the pregnancy.

thought he could change Pat's mind at that stage he was wrong. She went to see her son-in-law and daughter that weekend and came back to Raymond saying, 'I just took one look at their faces, their excitement, and that's what I'm going to do.'

For the unhappy Karen there was now hope. When her depression over being barren was at its deepest she had decided to confront the problem head on. With a friend she had started aerobics classes and exercise sessions for pregnant women at a small hall in the same complex as Raymond and Pat's shop off the town's high street. There she would counsel girls about breast-feeding, about looking after their new babies and how to keep fit during pregnancy. 'It helped me come to terms with my situation,' says Karen today. 'Instead of just bottling up my feelings I could talk about motherhood and help other people.'

It was a particularly courageous choice of occupation under the rather sad circumstances. And, although it made Karen less miserable, she was still not entirely the young woman of two years before. 'You could see the strain on my daughter even when Alcino Junior was two years old. Before she lost her uterus she was a bubbly person, bubbling all the time. Now she was quite flat,' remembers Raymond.

Then Pat came back to Tzaneen with her proposal. 'It was as though we had our daughter back again,' says Raymond. 'She became her old buoyant self and was very, very positive about Pat carrying the child.' Karen, despite all the doubts and difficulties to come, was sure this was going to be the solution to her problems.

Chapter 3

The craving for babies among the childless is as old as time itself. The married women of ancient Rome and Greece carried votive tablets shaped like genitals to their altars, beseeching the gods to grant them fertility. Stone-age tribesmen in Austria prayed to the 'Venus of Willendorf', a small, strange sexual idol that is one of the oldest human statues. And the tribes of Africa still ward off barrenness with amulets, masks and fertility dolls.

Today we have vastly more effective techniques to help couples have babies, techniques that, while their use may be highly emotive in our society, are a tribute to the incredible advances of medicine. And in the West, with one in nine couples of childbearing age unable to conceive easily or maintain a pregnancy, the demands on doctors to use modern science to make babies are increasing.

Baby fever is being fuelled by the number of women delaying their pregnancies into their 30s while they pursue careers. In America today four times as many women are having their first child between the ages of 30 and 34 as in 1967, although the female reproductive capacity begins to decline after the age of 24. In Britain and Europe the story is the same.

Doctors also cite the IUD – a plastic coil inserted close to the cervix to prevent pregnancy – as having increased infertility problems. The intrauterine device was widely used in the late 1960s and 1970s by women worried about the dangers of the contraceptive pill. But the IUD has been shown to relate to the widespread incidence of pelvic inflammatory disease, an often unrealized barrier to women conceiving.

And in this fast-moving world men too are helping to push up the infertility figures. Researchers in America and England estimate that 30 to 40 per cent of conception problems involve the husband alone. Male sexual weaknesses include impotence, accounting for 15 per cent of infertility, and a low sperm count caused by stress, drugs or alcohol, too many hot baths, and even excessive exercise, like jogging. All are factors which often play a part in modern lifestyles but are a barrier to natural baby-making.

The result is that more and more couples are prepared to go to endless lengths to overcome infertility and bring a baby into their lives. They will undergo the most uncomfortable and time-consuming tests, the most humiliating of examinations, and embark on lengthy medical programmes to conceive successfully. Their eagerness for it all to work is often accentuated by the fact that the woman's biological clock is running out of time. These couples are paying the price for waiting.

Men and women faced with infertility may feel cursed but they should also feel lucky. For all around them now are options, some frighteningly reminiscent of *Brave New World*, which will help them bring home the baby they want so much.

It was a decade ago that the miracles of modern science produced the world's first test-tube baby, Louise Brown. Now many babies across the globe, with America and Australia leading the race, have been conceived in a laboratory dish exactly like Louise. It is a process that is known as *in-vitro* (in-glass) fertilization. Louise was the first child in history to be conceived outside her mother's body, and consequently her birth made headlines. London's *Daily Mail*, which bought the exclusive rights to her story, trumpeted her arrival in the world exclaiming, 'It's a

Girl'. Publishing the first picture of the baby, the newspaper declared: 'And here she is . . . The Lovely Louise.' In America the *New York Post* said Louise, born in the down-to-earth British mill town of Oldham in Lancashire, was, 'The Tiny Miracle'.

Although her arrival was variously deemed to be a medical breakthrough, an ethical mistake and the beginning of a new and frightening age of genetic manipulation, the test-tube pioneers who masterminded the birth, Dr Patrick Steptoe and physiologist Dr Robert Edwards, became folk heroes. Within hours of Louise being born the two collaborators were besieged with requests for help from childless women who wanted test-tube babies.

There is no doubt that the birth of this baby, daughter of John Brown, a 38-year-old truck driver for British Rail in Bristol, and his wife, Lesley, 31, was a landmark for all childless couples. Lesley's blocked Fallopian tubes had been removed, and her husband had found the money to pay for the *in-vitro* fertilization after winning £750 on the football pools.

Steptoe and Edwards achieved their breakthrough by perfecting a technique that is still the basis of all *in-vitro* fertilizations. Although by 1977 they had succeeded in removing and fertilizing more than 80 eggs in glass test tubes and then implanting them back in the would-be mothers' wombs, none had survived more than a few months. But at the time when Lesley Brown was ready to conceive the two men had successfully adapted their technique.

Lesley Brown was given hormone treatment to stimulate her egg production before she made the crucial visit to Dr Kershaw's Cottage Hospital, in Oldham, Lancashire, for the actual conception of her child. Operating in the quaintly named institution's white-tiled surgical theatre, Dr Steptoe extracted an egg from his patient, using a laparoscope, a piece of equipment he helped to pioneer. The foot-long tube, used now in many *in-vitro* egg collections, is equipped with its own eye-piece and internal lighting and is inserted through a small slit in a woman's abdomen to select a ripening egg. A suction needle then removes the egg from her ovaries.

Dr Edwards then placed the egg in a small glass jar, where it was fertilized with John Brown's sperm and transferred to a nutrient solution to develop. The researchers monitored the egg as it divided into two, four and finally, after more than 50 hours, into eight cells.

This was the important moment, when they implanted the eight-cell embryo into Lesley Brown without waiting for it to develop further outside her body, as they had always done before. Previously they had copied nature, where the egg is normally fertilized within the woman's Fallopian tube and has multiplied into 64 or more cells by the time it reaches the womb. However, new research in 1977, using rhesus monkeys, had revealed that an embryo still at the two-cell stage could survive successfully inside the uterus.

But Steptoe and Edwards had few precedents to guide them in their pioneering of the test-tube baby technique. The first report of an *in-vitro* fertilization came in 1936 when Dr Gregory Pincus of Harvard University had united a rabbit egg and sperm. In 1961 Dr Daniele Patrucci of the University of Bologna, Italy, shocked the world with a claim – backed up by documentary film – that he had fertilized 20 separate human eggs outside the womb in a glass dish. Yet at that time the prospect of test-tube babies seemed so bizarre, even to scientists, that the research was greeted with outraged disbelief and subsequently ignored.

Since 1978 and Louise's birth by Caesarian section, an enormous amount of research has gone into improving the procedures involved. At the East Virginia Medical School, Norfolk, USA, which houses the oldest *in-vitro* clinic in America, doctors are now claiming a pregnancy rate of 31 per cent, although some of these pregnancies do result in miscarriage. There Dr Howard Jones, who founded the clinic, admits, 'A lot depends on whether a good egg meets a good sperm, rather like going to Las Vegas.'

In 1985 there were more than 300 medical reports published on human *in-vitro* fertilizations and the number of clinics offering test-tube baby techniques had multiplied. In Britain there are now 25 centres giving the service and 59 are officially registered in the United States. Australia and nearly every country in Western Europe have *in-vitro* centres too.

In Britain the overall success rate for *in-vitro* fertilization is around 11.5 per cent, which means that for each couple undergoing the full treatment there is just over a one in ten chance of the woman becoming pregnant.

The chances of a couple taking a baby home are even lower. Only one in 11 treatments result in a live child being born. However, some clinics are more successful than others, with a rate of live birth of up to 30 per cent. Doctors still do not know why an apparently healthy embryo is three times less likely to develop if it starts out in a laboratory saucer rather than in the womb of a woman who has conceived naturally.

The average couple in Britain currently makes three attempts at *in-vitro* fertilization, costing from £5,000 to £6,000 in total. One couple has undergone 14 attempts and is still trying to conceive the baby they have always wanted. People go without a car or foreign holidays and will take out a second mortgage to pay for treatment. 'Many, especially those who rush into this without full investigation about what is really wrong, end up a lot sadder, a bit wiser, and much poorer,' said one doctor.

But for *in-vitro* fertilization to be the solution for childless couples, the woman must be capable both of producing an egg and carrying the child in her womb. If she has no womb, or fails to ovulate, then the test-tube technique on its own is useless.

It is these women, for whom *in-vitro* fertilization is impossible, who have been turning to surrogacy in a last-ditch attempt to have a baby. Surrogacy, of course, is not a new idea and throughout history infertile women have resorted to procuring other women to carry their husband's child. The Old Testament has several examples, notably Sarah who said to Abraham: 'Behold now the Lord has prevented me from bearing children; go into my maid . . . that I may obtain children by her . . . and he went into Hagar,' who then bore the unfortunate Ishmael.

To date there have been more than 600 surrogate births in America where a woman has carried a baby, created by the insemination of her egg by sperm of the husband of an infertile couple. Most of these have been commercial arrangements. Some have ended in disaster, as amply illustrated by the Baby M trial in New Jersey, where the surrogate mother, Mary Beth Whitehead, has fought to keep the daughter she bore for Elizabeth and William Stern (see page 67). But the pioneer of surrogacy agencies, Harriett Blankfield, who runs Infertility Associates in the United States, insists:

> The percentage of arrangements that run into problems is very small. Surrogacy is the last alternative for many people. They have already gone through surgery, *in-vitro* fertilization and often an adoption attempt. But there are not enough adoptable babies.

Britain's first commercial surrogate mother was Kim Cotton, who gave birth to a daughter, known later in legal parlance as Baby Cotton, in the Victoria Maternity Hospital, Barnet, North London, on 4 January 1985. In the April of the previous year Kim Cotton had been artificially inseminated, in the bedroom of her family home, with the sperm of a man she had never met. This man, who remained anonymous throughout the uproar that followed the birth, and his infertile wife had paid an agreed fee of £6,500 to Mrs Cotton for carrying the baby.

It was like any other surrogacy deal up to that time. Baby Cotton was created from the egg of Kim Cotton which was then fertilized by the anonymous fee-paying partner in the contract. This man's infertile wife, who would become Baby Cotton's mother, had absolutely no biological or genetic input into the child that was to become hers.

After the birth of Baby Cotton, Barnet Social Services Committee met in an emergency session to discuss the future of the little girl. The Committee wanted to determine if the future parents, believed to come from America, were suitable to take care of Baby Cotton.

And a few days after the baby's arrival there was a High Court hearing to look at the same issue. Baby Cotton had meanwhile been made a Ward of Court and taken into a place of safety to await the outcome of the High Court judgement, which was eventually announced on Monday 14 January, ten days after the birth.

The judge, Mr Justice Latey, deemed the natural father of Baby Cotton and his wife to be a 'warm, caring, sensible couple' who would give the baby a good home. The judge said that Baby Cotton's birth certificate would be sealed and by court order the parents' identity would not be revealed.

The couple, who lived abroad, had already left Britain with the baby over the previous weekend. Their departure was kept secret, the whereabouts of Baby Cotton never made public.

Now laboratory baby-making has allowed further advances and there have been the first 'host womb' surrogacies. In these the egg from a woman who has no womb can be fertilized by her own husband's sperm, using the *in-vitro* techniques. Then that tiny embryo created in a test tube is placed in the womb of a surrogate mother for her to carry to term. Genetically the surrogate mother is a complete outsider, simply an incubator and nothing more.

Suddenly couples who are unable to conceive will have the chance of having their own children, as long as the wife can produce her own eggs. And although it is a controversial move down the path of medical experimentation, it is expected to become a very satisfactory solution for the infertile.

Dr Cecil Michelow, the doctor in charge of the surrogate grandmother, Pat Anthony, believes host womb surrogacies are the way forward.

It is ideal because the embryo that is transferred to grow inside the surrogate belongs biologically to the infertile couple.

The surrogate is only allowing her womb to be used as the incubator for the embryo that is being placed in it. The surrogate is not actually giving any part of herself.

But the chances of host womb surrogacies succeeding are rare, because of the complicated process involved in preparing the surrogate for reception of the alien embryo.

'The synchronization of the monthly cycles of the surrogate with the woman who is giving the egg is vitally important. The surrogate and biological mother must be made to ovulate together so the host womb is absolutely ready to accept the embryo,' explains Dr Michelow.

The quest for a child, carried by a surrogate but biologically their own, is now the business of many couples. Although it has never happened in Britain, host womb births are the beginning of a brighter, less complex future for the infertile. In the United States a teacher of 41 and a 30-year-old mental health worker have undergone endless tests to try to achieve a surrogate pregnancy.

The teacher is Norma Peters, from Longview, Washington, who was born without a uterus, a condition that occurs naturally in about one in every 1,000 women. Although she and her husband Bob, aged 45, have adopted two children during their barren 23-year-old marriage, they still hope for their own baby.

After Louise Brown was born in 1978, the couple started to contact doctors and scientists in England, Australia, Canada and the United States. They wanted to know whether an embryo fertilized using the test-tube technique could then be implanted in another woman. They were told by one shocked doctor that it was a wild idea. Others replied that nothing like that was yet on the infertility agenda.

Last year Norma Peters was introduced to Alexis Brown, the Californian mental health worker and mother of three, who after being sterilized 'missed being pregnant'. 'I love to feel babies fluttering in my tummy, but I don't want any more children of my own.' So far there are three embryos, created from Norma's eggs and Bob's sperm, waiting and frozen at minus 196° centigrade in a special freezer at the Southern California Fertility Institute. But, because Alexis's hormone levels are not sufficiently high for doctors to prepare her womb lining for the implantation, the embryo transfer has been delayed.

Norma and Bob Peters are still hopeful but Dr William Karow, director of the Institute, puts the chances of this host womb venture succeeding at only two or three per cent.

There are other options too, courtesy of new technology, including egg or embryo donation which helps women who are able to carry children but have no eggs. By 1987 more than 30 infertile women in Britain had been helped by this method, which has been given guarded approval by the watchdog of ethics in test-tube baby techniques, the Warnock Committee. The wife who has no eggs receives them from another woman, either donated anonymously or from a female relative, and they are fertilized by her husband's sperm before being implanted in her womb.

Last November 30-year-old Ann Johnson gave birth to twins at a private hospital in Nottingham, although her ovaries had stopped functioning. Ann, who had known for years she could not conceive, had been given the egg from her sister Sandra, which was then fertilized by her own husband Steve before being implanted into her own hormone-primed body. She decided to go ahead with the treatment after a handful of other women in Britain had successfully used their sisters' eggs.

Although the babies, Danielle and Carla, who grew in Ann's womb were genetically Sandra's, Ann went through the pregnancy and said she felt psychologically the true mother, experiencing the mother-and-baby bonding at birth. 'Carrying a child is a big part of having a baby,' she said. 'Sandra and I have similar personalities and even looks, and I couldn't have got any closer to having my own child.'

And Sandra added:

> I suppose I do feel closer to the babies, but not enough to interfere. They are just my nieces. Children are always asking about their family and it will be much better to be able to tell them the truth when they grow up. Unlike an anonymous donation of an egg we know their whole background.

An egg donation within the family has other advantages. Ann's children will have the same biological grandparents as they would if they were entirely her own and Steve's.

For unexplained infertility there is another route forward with gamete interfallopian transfer, known as GIFT, where the eggs and sperm are brought together outside the woman's body and then immediately put back into a Fallopian tube to create a more natural atmosphere than a test tube for development of the egg and conception. This is a method that can be twice as successful as *in-vitro* fertilization, largely because a woman who is suitable for the GIFT procedure must have one healthy tube so her chances of pregnancy are higher before she even starts.

When we look back at the last decade, and the developments which have followed from the birth of Louise Brown, it is remarkable how swift the progress has been. Until then only rats, mice and rabbits had undergone successful test-tube fertilization, with no experimentation at all on man's closest relatives, monkeys and apes. Apparently Steptoe and Edwards were so confident they were on the right path that they simply skipped experimentation with the non-human primates.

But research on animals is vital, for it foreshadows the future. Now, after treatment with hormones, a genetically superior cow can be inseminated artificially so she produces as many as 16 embryos. These are then flushed from the cow's womb and reimplanted in inferior cows, which carry the calves to term. The result is a far more rapid improvement of the breed than unaided nature permits, but a human parallel would have horrifying implications.

Animal researchers are also slowly moving towards a true test-tube baby. Even back in the 1960s Canadian scientists had managed to nurture lamb embryos withdrawn prematurely from their mothers. Placed in plastic containers, the lamb embryos were bathed in a solution similar to amniotic fluid from the womb, and linked to a mechanical blood-circulation system, rather like a heart-lung machine.

The lambs survived the artificial environment and were then reborn, 'decanted', as Aldous Huxley termed it in *Brave New World*. At the Johns Hopkins University in America mice embryos have been kept alive in a petri dish or test tube for half their typical 19-day gestation period. And it has to be recognized that experts will soon have the technology to produce artificial wombs that will take test-tube humans from conception to birth.

Couples in which only the husband is infertile are also still using artificial insemination, where the woman is given the sperm of an anonymous donor, as the solution to their childlessness. Roxanne Feldschuh, co-director of Idant in New York, the world's largest sperm bank, says, 'Married couples want two things from a donor, a resemblance to the husband and intelligence'. Increasingly, sperm banks are freezing supplies so that a couple who want more than one child can go back several years later for a second insemination from the same donor. The resulting children are true siblings.

The freezing of eggs and embryos has been perfected during the 1980s, allowing even more flexibility and choice for the childless. In March 1984, Mary Wright underwent fertility treatment at the Bourn Hall Clinic, under Professor Robert Edwards and Dr Patrick Steptoe, and produced ten eggs. Mrs Wright, 35, had two children by her first husband and was then sterilized. She subsequently married again and wanted more children. So Edwards and Steptoe proceeded with the treatment, and when it failed to achieve a pregnancy, Mrs Wright and her husband Phillip's six remaining fertilized eggs were stored at sub-zero temperatures.

In January 1985, two of the embryos were thawed and implanted in Mrs Wright. Nine months later her daughter Amy was born. It was just over a year later, in July 1986, that she returned to see if 'the miracle of Amy could be repeated'. And in 1987, 18 months later, her 'time-warp twin', Elizabeth, came into the world. High-tech embryology had won its-way, as Steptoe commented: 'Amy and Elizabeth are unique. They were conceived in one batch of Mrs Wright's eggs and with one donation of her husband's sperm.'

Freezing means that women in danger of losing their eggs or ovaries through disease, infection or premature ageing can literally sidestep what the future holds for them. Their eggs can be fertilized by their husband's sperm and held in frozen readiness for implantation into their wombs at any time they select. Doctors are now also predicting that women with no reproductive problems at all may start using egg or embryo preservation as a matter of social convenience in family planning.

The question is: to what lengths will infertile couples go in their battle to achieve parenthood? A survey of patients attending an *in-vitro* fertilization programme in Australia showed the majority would have opted for adoption if it had been possible. Of the third who took part in the study, 63 per cent said they would have considered adopting a normal baby in Australia itself, and 36 per would have been open to the idea of adopting a child from another country. That is an indication that substitute methods of becoming parents have not been rejected outright, and indeed if there were more children available for adoption perhaps the test-tube baby revolution would never have progressed so speedily.

Abortion, society's acceptance of single parenthood and increased infertility have all served to make adoption increasingly difficult. In America it is estimated that three million couples are now looking to adopt and there are only 50,000 healthy white infants available. Private adoptions, where a lawyer rather than a recognized agency is used as the middleman, are increasing. And in Britain and Europe couples are travelling to the Third World nations, like South Korea, Thailand and Chile, to 'buy' babies for themselves.

Society may not be ready for the tremendous advances of medical science but technology has provided hope for the childless as never before. As one *in-vitro* patient recalls:

> The sorrow of infertility for a happily married couple can be compared to the sorrow of bereavement. The 'funeral' starts in the hospital out-patient clinic when the couple learns the results of 'tests'. The mourning continues for years with occasional surges of hope that a miracle may happen.
>
> Now, thankfully, more of those miracles are possible.

Chapter 4

Dr Cecil Michelow, the distinguished doctor who had practised as a Johannesburg gynaecologist for more than 30 years, first heard of the Tzaneen grandmother who wished to carry her own grandchild at the end of June 1986. It was then, during a busy morning, that the internal telephone buzzed in his consulting rooms at the Vita Lab fertility clinic, and waiting to speak to him was his excited younger colleague, Dr Johan Van Der Wat.

Van Der Wat, who had his surgery on the floor below Michelow's at the Park Lane Clinic, got on well with the respected Jewish doctor and he made an extraordinary request to him. Would Michelow, and his Vita Lab partners, Dr Joel Bernstein and Dr Merwyn Jacobson, help a 47-year-old woman to become the surrogate mother for her own barren daughter's baby? This grandmother, explained Van Der Wat, had visited him three weeks before and they had talked of the possibility of her becoming a surrogate. 'I sent her home to discuss it with her family and now she is persisting she wants to go ahead,' he told Michelow. 'She is very determined, very certain about it all. I thought you might be prepared to take on the challenge.'

Michelow did want the challenge, and he shared Van Der Wat's commitment to 'making babies' for women who were childless. He and his artist wife had brought up three children and he rated the joys of parenthood highly. And now that Vita Lab, the fertility clinic he had helped found, was three years old, this was just the sort of case that he and his partners should be taking on.

Just before the Vita Lab was started in 1983 Michelow and Bernstein had spent a month in Australia as guests of the infertility unit at the Royal Women's Hospital in Melbourne. They worked with the laboratory technicians, assisted in cases and helped the unit celebrate its bicentenary. For the Royal Women's Hospital had pioneered *in-vitro* fertilization in Australia and Michelow and Bernstein were there to learn everything the Melbourne unit could tell them about test-tube technology.

When the two doctors returned to South Africa they built the Vita Lab, which was identical to the one at the Royal Women's Hospital, and in July 1985 they admitted their first patient. From the outset the Vita Lab team declared themselves prepared to help the most hopeless of cases, even women who were running out of time and had reached 40. This Pat Anthony, mused Michelow after he finished speaking to Van Der Wat, would probably never be able to conceive, but he was willing to try.

> Van Der Wat told me that Karen Ferreira-Jorge had always wanted a family of four or five and personally I could understand why she was so unhappy. I suppose critics would protest she should have been content with one baby but that didn't bother me. Van Der Wat said that the proposed surrogate was then 47 but I decided it was an exciting and interesting case so I told him OK.

But after speaking to his partners, Bernstein and Jacobson, who were eager to go ahead, Dr Michelow sought advice from one of South Africa's leading legal experts on surrogacy, Professor S.A. Strauss at the University of South Africa, half an hour away from Johannesburg, in Pretoria.

Professor Strauss was away from the university in southwest Africa and it was not until a month later that Michelow was first able to explain the unusual case of the shopkeeper's wife from Tzaneen and her desperately miserable daughter. Strauss was immediately enthusiastic. 'He said it would be an ideal case,' recalls Michelow, 'because the granny would be acting purely as a surrogate womb for her daughter and son-in-law's embryo. So that when these babies were born there would be firstly no money changing hands and no problem as far as giving back the child.'

Strauss encouraged the doctor: 'Go ahead, you have my blessing and I think you are going to make a lot of people very happy.' But he insisted that Vita Lab made a contract with Pat Anthony and her family to safeguard the doctors, the same sort of contract that every *in-vitro* fertilization patient at the Park Lane Clinic is asked to sign.

'This simply outlines the treatment the patient will receive, that there are certain risks involved in test-tube technology though these appear to be the same as in normal pregnancy, and that the doctors cannot guarantee that the end result of going in the *in-vitro* programme will be a baby.'

But because of the unique nature of Pat Anthony's case, the doctors and their lawyers prepared another legal document, a contract between Pat, Karen and Alcino. It read: 'This is to confirm that Mrs Anthony has agreed to act as the surrogate mother to the embryo transfer as a result of the fertilization of her daughter's ovum by her son-in-law's sperm.'

More importantly it added: 'Mrs Anthony has agreed to give the baby of such treatment back to her daughter and son-in-law who are the child's genetic parents.'

By the time the legal documents had been drawn up and signed it was the middle of August, and Michelow was growing concerned that the grandmother he had not yet met would reach the menopause before she was given the chance of becoming a surrogate mother.

The thing that came into my mind after talking to Van Der Wat was the age of the granny, for we know that fertility starts dropping really dramatically after the age of 40.

We knew that Pat Anthony had a good record of fertility, because she had produced two kids before, but we realized that even highly productive women do lose their fertility as they get older. Yet I remembered in the old days we used to have patients coming in with their 10th, 11th and 12th child up to the age of 49, although here in Johannesburg there has never been a pregnant mother of 50 or more.

When Pat had undergone tests earlier in the year they had shown she would soon have the change of life. And it was essential if she was to be a successful surrogate for her body still to be fertile, still ready to receive and hold an embryo in her womb. Michelow explains: 'When I first saw Pat on 26 August 1986, she was 47 and very close to her last period, so speed was of the essence here and we didn't feel so hopeful about it. But the point is the challenge was presented and we thought we must give it a try before it is too late.'

The day was a Tuesday and Karen remembers how she and her mother walked into the Vita Lab for the first time. 'We sat down in front of Dr Michelow and he joked and said: "Now who is going to be the surrogate here?" Straightaway the friendly atmosphere of the whole place, of the doctors and the nursing sisters, impressed us so much.'

The doctors started treatment the same day, for the medical problems were mighty. Ensuring that any implantation of Karen's fertilized eggs into her mother was successful meant perfecting the synchronization of the two women's monthly cycles. Both mother and daughter would have to be made to ovulate at precisely the same time of the month so that when Karen's eggs were produced Pat's womb would be receptive to the embryos being put in.

To complicate matters the doctors had to discover exactly when Karen ovulated, no easy task because she had had no period since the hysterectomy to give guidelines. For two months they struggled while Pat and Karen travelled back and forth between Tzaneen and the Park Lane Clinic for tests and more tests. Every morning in Tzaneen, the moment she woke up, Alcino would put a thermometer into Karen's mouth to take her temperature.

If her temperature had dropped and then risen dramatically it would indicate she had ovulated, but week after week nothing happened. Suddenly Karen had stopped ovulating. She remembers those days:

> You have to put the thermometer in your mouth the minute you wake up, you're not allowed to pick up your arms, move your hands, talk, smoke or do anything. If you have a disturbed night, as I was doing practically every night with Alcino Junior, then it influences the temperature. In the end the chart I kept showed I had ovulated when I hadn't ovulated. We were in a muddle.

So in early December the Vita Lab doctors decided to put Pat and Karen on the contraceptive pill, one which was oestrogen-based. It was a simple way of controlling their cycles and for 28 days, throughout the family Christmas in Tzaneen, the two women took their pill daily. When the packet finished both Pat and Karen started their new cycle on exactly the same day. It was 7 January.

The Vita Lab plan was to implant Karen's eggs into her mother on the 18th day of the cycle, Saturday, 24 January. Both women would, according to Dr Michelow's calculations, have ovulated two days earlier on 22 January. It was a tense time and Pat, although still enthusiastic, had suffered through the Christmas at Tzaneen as the contraceptive pill she was taking made her feel sick, and no one but Raymond, Karen and Alcino knew why she was feeling ill.

On 9 January Karen was given a hormone stimulant, like women on the test-tube baby programme who go on to carry their own child, to make sure she would ovulate and that the eggs she managed to produce would not evaporate into her system too soon. Three days later Pat was also given hormones to ensure she ovulated well that month.

Day 14 of their cycles was crucial for the success of the daring operation. At ten o'clock that night, 20 January, both Karen and Pat went to the Park Lane Clinic to receive injections to further encourage their ovulation together in exactly 36 hours' time. But already the doctors were hopeful, for their tests showed that Karen had at least 11 follicles inside her, which would each produce an egg.

At eight o'clock on the morning of 22 January Karen drove to the clinic from a friend's house in Johannesburg for the removal of her eggs. It was 34 hours to the minute after the last injection and precisely two hours before she actually ovulated. The timing was designed so Karen's eggs were still attached to the follicles, in one place and ready to be picked up. Two hours later, when ovulation happened, they would have dispersed into her Fallopian tubes, making it impossible for doctors to find them.

With Dr Michelow at her side Karen was wheeled into the operating theatre and put under general anaesthetic for ten minutes while the eggs were taken from her. There were 11 in all although, remarkably, she had produced 22 that month.

Alcino, who had been away in the country on a bachelor fishing trip, kept an appointment at the Park Lane Clinic that morning too. He gave a sperm sample and as the eggs were taken from Karen the laboratory team started their work. First they prepared his sperm by incubating it in a culture medium for six hours, which gave the sperm a better capacity to fertilize the eggs.

The eggs were also placed in this culture medium for six hours to allow them to mature. Then 100,000 sperm were put into each of the 11 little laboratory saucers containing an egg. It was two o'clock in the afternoon and it wouldn't be until the following day that the Vita Lab doctors would be able to tell if fertilization was taking place. That would be at ten o'clock on Friday morning, or Day 17.

'It was obvious on that Friday that the eggs had been fertilized, but we had to wait another 24 hours to find out if they were dividing into cells as they should do. We hoped to see two, three, four or five cells, or even more,' explains Dr Michelow. 'On the Saturday morning the news was good, we were all delighted. And we then selected the best embryos ready to transfer them into Pat. Ten of the 11 had developed.'

Doctors, even those at the forefront of test-tube technology and fertility work, have no really failsafe system of choosing those 'best' eggs. As Michelow explains:

> Technology still isn't advanced enough for a proper system to have been devised. We look at the moment for an evenness of the cells, a good appearance, an overall consistency. These, I have to say, are crude methods at the moment because we just don't know which are the better eggs, or which are going to become the better embryos.

Pat had also produced an egg 48 hours earlier, just one according to the doctors. And it was important that Karen's eggs, surrounded by Alcino's sperm, were not implanted into her until this had died. 'We had to make absolutely sure that his sperm did not meet his mother-in-law's egg,' said Michelow. But an egg will only live for 24 hours and the one released in Pat on the Thursday had died on the Friday.

It was 12 noon on Saturday when Karen and her mother arrived back at the clinic to hear from Sister Sharon Preddy, an assistant to the doctors, that the historic implant of four eggs into Pat's womb could go ahead. Pat, in one of the hospital green gowns, was hustled up the stairs of the clinic to the theatre because she had booked in under her own name, and was afraid her secret would be discovered.

Normally at the Park Lane Clinic an embryo transfer, after a test-tube fertilization, takes place with the husband at the wife's theatre bedside. It is a way of involving the husband in the creation of his children, a way of breaking down the barriers that this 'Brave New World' technology must inevitably bring between a man and a woman.

But Pat went to the theatre on her own. She lay there as the four healthy embryos fertilized by her son-in-law were placed gently inside her body. With a small catheter they were inserted through her cervix and put at the entrance of her womb. It was only a ten-minute operation but the final stage of five months of preparation.

When Pat was wheeled back to the ward to rest she was instructed to lie with her feet up for two hours. She recalls:

> I didn't take any chances. I lay in that hospital bed with my feet up for four hours just to make absolutely sure. I was worried that nothing would happen. I wanted it all to work so desperately for Karen's sake. She really believed in what the doctors were doing and I just prayed that one of those embryos would be conceived in me.

And this remarkable lady, who seemed to spend so little time thinking of herself or her sacrifice, did another extraordinary thing that day. She had been an habitual smoker for most of her adult life. Every day in Tzaneen she would buy three packets of 20 and puff her way through them. 'I loved a cigarette, just like Raymond does,' she explains. 'But from the moment I came out of the operating theatre after the implant I gave up for good.'

Karen says,

> I was amazed because she used to smoke 60 a day and she stopped just like that. I really admired her for doing it because I never thought she would. I had said I was worried about her smoking if she became pregnant for me and Alcino. But I didn't really put any pressure on my mother. It was her decision and her decision alone. But I was very pleased and proud of her.

All night Pat lay at the Park Lane Clinic and the next morning Karen and Alcino came to collect her. Already Pat says she felt pregnant and she told her family so. 'But although she kept insisting she felt something we didn't respond much,' says Karen. 'We just privately hoped she was not getting too excited or anxious because the disappointment for her, as well as us, would have been terrible to face.'

In fact Pat's chances of pregnancy were not good at all. By putting four eggs into Pat the doctors hoped to improve the odds of one surviving. Dr Michelow explains now:

> We only ever thought that we would achieve one successful pregnancy. The statistics show that if one egg is implanted in a woman there is a ten per cent chance of a pregnancy.
>
> If two embryos are implanted then it becomes 15 to 17 per cent, and when three are put in her the odds improve dramatically, up to 23 per cent.

With four embryos the chances can improve slightly, but procreation pioneers across the world agree that there is no point in putting any more embryos into a woman. The statistics for successful pregnancies reveal that an implantation of five or six eggs achieves the same results as if four eggs are placed in the womb.

'We had the odd twin pregnancy before when we put in three or four embryos and that is why we decided to use four with Pat,' explains Dr Michelow. 'We put them in for another good reason, because of her age more than anything else and the fact we didn't really know what her fertility was like.'

No one knew then that all four of those eggs were to take, and three were to survive to birth. 'Either our laboratory conditions at the time were superb, or Pat was highly receptive, much more so than we could have dreamed. Most important, possibly, was that the embryos were those of a young couple, or a couple with proven fertility,' says Dr Michelow.

But one thing is certain, as the doctors and nurses waited for the days to go by before they would discover if the fragile Pat Anthony was pregnant, they only ever thought of one baby. 'In fact that would have been ideal, that was all we were ever trying to achieve. And at the time it was everything that Pat, Karen and Alcino wanted. A brother or sister for Alcino,' recalls Michelow.

And Dr Jacobson, the bachelor 40-year-old who made up the partnership, is still incredulous. 'There we had a lady of advanced age acting as a surrogate. Her ovaries were getting tired, she was nearing the menopause and even after being given hormone stimulants her ovulation was very poor. One baby would have been exceptional at the end of it.'

And what the doctors didn't know was how nearly Pat had given up under the strain of the hospital tests and the amount of pills and injections she was taking during the months running up to the implant. Raymond provided a shoulder for her to cry on and Pat told him that if she wasn't pregnant by February she might not carry on, even for Karen's sake.

Raymond recalls:

> The pills she was taking were making her nauseous, uncomfortable and tired, and it was this that actually got her in the end. She said to me, 'God, if I have to go through another month of this I may give up'. But thankfully then came the news she was pregnant.

At the time Pat and Karen never realized how remote were the chances of the surrogacy actually happening. It is only today, with the babies beyond their first birthday, that they realize the brilliance of the astonishing medical miracle. And this devout family also think the doctors were God's handmaidens.

Raymond explains: 'I think that God made triplets when nobody was dreaming of that. It was his way of saying to Karen and Alcino that they should have the four children they originally wanted.'

As for Pat, so certain she was pregnant from 24 hours

after the implant, and hoping against hope that she would never have to undergo another month on the fertility programme, she prayed as she has always done. And ten days after the four little embryos were placed in her, the period doctors had expected to come along never happened. Pat Anthony was on her way to becoming a surrogate mother for her own grandchildren.

Chapter 5

Pat kept an important appointment at the Park Lane Clinic exactly one month after the implant into her body of the tiny embryos created in a laboratory dish.

Even though it was her birthday, she had noted the time of 3.15 in the afternoon of Monday, 23 February 1987 in her diary, and ringed it in pencil. Pat was nervous when Karen and Alcino, who had travelled by car from Tzaneen, drove up to the clinic five minutes late. The couple had been delayed by shopping in the city's Carlton Centre for a new double bed.

But together the three walked into the basement rooms of Vita Lab on time, outwardly trying to look calm but each equally edgy about what they would soon discover. None of the family trio had time that afternoon to remember that it was exactly three years earlier when they had dined at the El Toro Steak House in Tzaneen as Karen started to have contractions before the birth of her first and only son.

In the Vita Lab that afternoon Sister Sharon Preddy was waiting for the very special patient. Although all the Vita Lab team reasoned that every infertility case was of the same merit, Pat Anthony's courage and dignity had caught their attention and both doctors and nurses admired what she was trying to do for her barren daughter.

Sister Sharon gently told Karen and Alcino to help themselves to a cup of coffee from the automatic machine and wait in Dr Michelow's empty consulting rooms. Then she guided Pat on her own through to the scan room, where the white-coated Dr Michelow switched on the machine and asked Pat to lie on the little bunk nearby.

Sister Sharon says: 'We decided Pat should be on her own, away from the rest of her family, when the scan was done. If we found there was no baby in there, she would need time alone to recover from her disappointment and prepare to break the news to Karen.'

Dr Michelow placed the sonar scan probe on Pat's naked stomach and the seconds ticked by as his eyes searched the screen for the first signs of human life. Then both he and Sister Sharon started talking at once. Amazingly, the doctor had found not one baby inside Pat, but two, their hearts beating healthily. 'Pat,' said the doctor steadily, 'I think Karen will be having twins in October.'

Pat remembers:

Very soon there was quite a crowd in the small scan room. The nurses all came in and were kissing each other and crying. Doctors Bernstein and Jacobson were called and they crammed in too. Everyone was slapping each other on the back. The three doctors were shaking everybody by the hand and congratulating themselves. They realized they had achieved something really fantastic.

Sister Sharon was the first to move. She ran out of the scan room and down the short corridor to Dr Michelow's surgery where Karen and Alcino were waiting. 'Come and see, quickly, there are twins,' she told them.

'We rushed to the scan room and Dr Michelow showed us the first little baby on the screen, then they moved to the second. For us it was the most wonderfully moving moment,' says Karen.

My mother was holding my hand and saying, 'Are you happy? Are you happy?' and then Dr Jacobson picked up the probe and started looking at the screen again. He moved the probe around a bit on my mother's tummy and suddenly he came across something else. He exclaimed: 'There are three darn babies in here!' and we just couldn't believe it. The atmosphere in that room was electric.

While, as Karen says in her soft South African accent, 'everyone was going nuts', Dr Jacobson was searching for the heart beat of the third little embryo. He couldn't find it that day, and it was only when everyone else had left the scan room that he was to warn Karen and Pat that this baby might not survive. By the time Pat came in for her next scan, this embryo in its little sac might have dissolved and disappeared.

Dr Michelow recalls that afternoon with perfect clarity.

We hoped Pat was pregnant but we knew the chances were remote. When I first looked on the scan screen and saw a baby I was thrilled because it confirmed that against pretty substantial odds she was expecting one. No one was more surprised than me to discover a second baby, and then a third.

Inside Pat the doctors also spotted a fourth sac, which seemed to be empty.

We weren't too happy about the idea of quads, especially inside a 48-year-old woman. But the fact that the sac was empty meant that the embryo had blighted some days before and stopped growing. The sac tissue would be reabsorbed, I told the family, and when the birth happened there would be no sign of it.

Dr Bernstein too was amazed that their patient was pregnant.

We were startled that she had conceived at all, let alone

had three. Under normal circumstances there would have been a 22 per cent chance of Pat conceiving one baby, but because of her age and a low sperm count from Alcino who had just been away on a bachelor fishing trip where there was quite a lot of drinking, we put the odds at between nought and 5 per cent.

Before that scan was taken there seemed to be only one person certain that Pat was pregnant. 'I realized I was expecting a baby a few days after the January implant, and well before the scan. I told Karen but I don't think the family really believed me,' says Pat.

'I felt queasy almost immediately and like many pregnant women I put on 12 pounds in three weeks. I just knew I was going to have a baby, although I was still nervous about the scan in case anything was wrong.'

The realization that Pat was expecting triplets sent the whole family into a state of shock. As they left the clinic in Junction Avenue that night the doctors told Pat that she must not travel back to Tzaneen. Instead she had to stay in Johannesburg for the rest of the pregnancy, eating well, sleeping well, and near at hand if there was an unexpected emergency.

When Pat rang Raymond from the clinic to tell him the extraordinary news he was waiting at the shop.

Up till then I had been a bit reticent about the whole business because I didn't think it could ever work. When they telephoned that day and told me there were three on the way I didn't believe Pat or Karen. I said, now come on man, don't play the fool over a thing like this. And it took some convincing for me to believe it.

He wonders now if the family would ever have gone through with the idea of Pat being the surrogate if they had ever in their wildest dreams thought it would be triplets. 'Carrying three was an extra health problem and I don't think I would have wished my wife to go on, even for Karen, if I had known.'

Alcino too was shocked. When Karen asked him outside the scan room if he was happy at the news late that afternoon, he admits,

> I lied to her. I said I am very, very pleased, but I wasn't at all. I was terrified, in fact. I was thinking now here we are with three babies and I don't know how we are going to handle it. It was only a week or so later that I convinced myself that we would manage.

Karen and Alcino drove back to Tzaneen, out in the Northern Transvaal, in the dark and in almost total silence — they were worried as well as excited at the prospect of this most unusual kind of parenthood. How would they explain in Tzaneen what had happened? What would they tell their friends, if anything at all? How could they keep one of the most unusual pregnancies in the world a secret as Pat had insisted it must be?

If Pat, normally so easy going, had been adamant about anything as the extraordinary surrogacy pact got underway, it was that her anonymity should be preserved. She was concerned about the reaction of the South African public to her pregnancy, the attitude of the government in a country not renowned for its broad-mindedness and the stance of the Dutch Reformed Church which dominated the thinking of so many leading Afrikaners in policy-making positions.

Pat, never a woman for show, wanted to go quietly ahead with the pregnancy and birth without the eyes of the world upon her. To her it was a family affair, an arrangement between a mother and her unhappy daughter. Nothing more. She explains:

> After the scan I planned to go back to Tzaneen and work in the shop for three or four months, until my tummy started to show. Then I had thought I would rent a small

flat in Johannesburg for the rest of the pregnancy.

When the birth happened I would hand the baby, or babies, over to Karen to take home to Tzaneen. She would tell people that she had found a surrogate mother overseas, even in Portugal where Alcino's parents now live, who had carried the child. I thought I could return to Tzaneen soon after as though nothing had happened.

Pat was also worried that the more ignorant would never understand how she was carrying her son-in-law's children. They might think, she reasoned, that she had slept with Alcino to conceive the babies, or that they were genetically hers and her son-in-law's. For a Roman Catholic who took her religion seriously, this would be a catastrophe.

Yet Pat's scheme to return to Tzaneen, and then disappear for the rest of the pregnancy, was impossible. Now she was carrying triplets and there would be no interlude before her small body started to swell. By three months into the pregnancy, she looked like a woman who had reached her sixth month. By her fifth month, Pat looked ready to give birth.

The day after the scan, Karen had promised Alcino Junior a proper party to celebrate his third birthday. The trip back from Tzaneen the night before had tired her, but she went ahead laying the tables on the patio with the help of her black housemaid, Sabena.

My friends all came with their babies and I was dying to tell somebody I was expecting triplets, except that my mother was acting as the incubator for them. I wanted to shout that by October I would be a mother again, three times over. But the family had agreed that I wasn't allowed to say one word, for my mother's sake.

While Pat began her stay in Johannesburg on doctor's orders, Raymond was to bear the brunt of the constant inquiries about his missing wife. Raymond, who thought his family were joking when they rang him from the Park

Lane Clinic to announce triplets were on the way, found it more and more difficult as day after day at his shop questions about Pat had to be sidestepped.

'By the end of March, five weeks after the scan, the people in Tzaneen began to say that Raymond and I had separated and that our marriage was on the rocks,' recalls Pat today. 'They couldn't understand why I was living in Johannesburg and he was still at the shop.'

When Raymond denied that he and Pat were permanently apart, the stories began to circulate about her having a serious disease, even cancer. 'I told some very close friends that Karen and Alcino had found themselves a surrogate mother, but I never said it was Pat away in Johannesburg. I just said Pat was having some medical check-ups,' he remembers.

Karen and Alcino confided the full story to a few friends as the weeks went by, including the couple they invited to supper in the middle of March. They were Joe and Magdelene Darvas, the Roman Catholic parents of South Africa's first ever test-tube baby, who lived in Tzaneen. Their daughter Dominique Darvas, now six, was born on 6 January 1982 at the Bourn Hall laboratory near Cambridge run by British fertility expert Dr Patrick Steptoe. Like Karen and Alcino, the Darvases had defied the Catholic Church's rulings on procreation and produced a little girl with all the help of medical technology.

That evening Joe and Magdelene listened as Alcino related how his mother-in-law wanted to keep this extraordinary episode in their lives secret. Alcino said he believed Pat's decision was the right one. 'We don't want the publicity,' he explained. 'We just want the babies to be normal and then get on with the rest of our lives.'

But Joe and Magdelene said something to make Alcino, and the listening Karen, change their minds. The Darvases related how after Dominique's unusual conception and birth they tried to keep their story quiet. But instead persistent South African journalists stalked them daily, then approached the Darvases at their house and

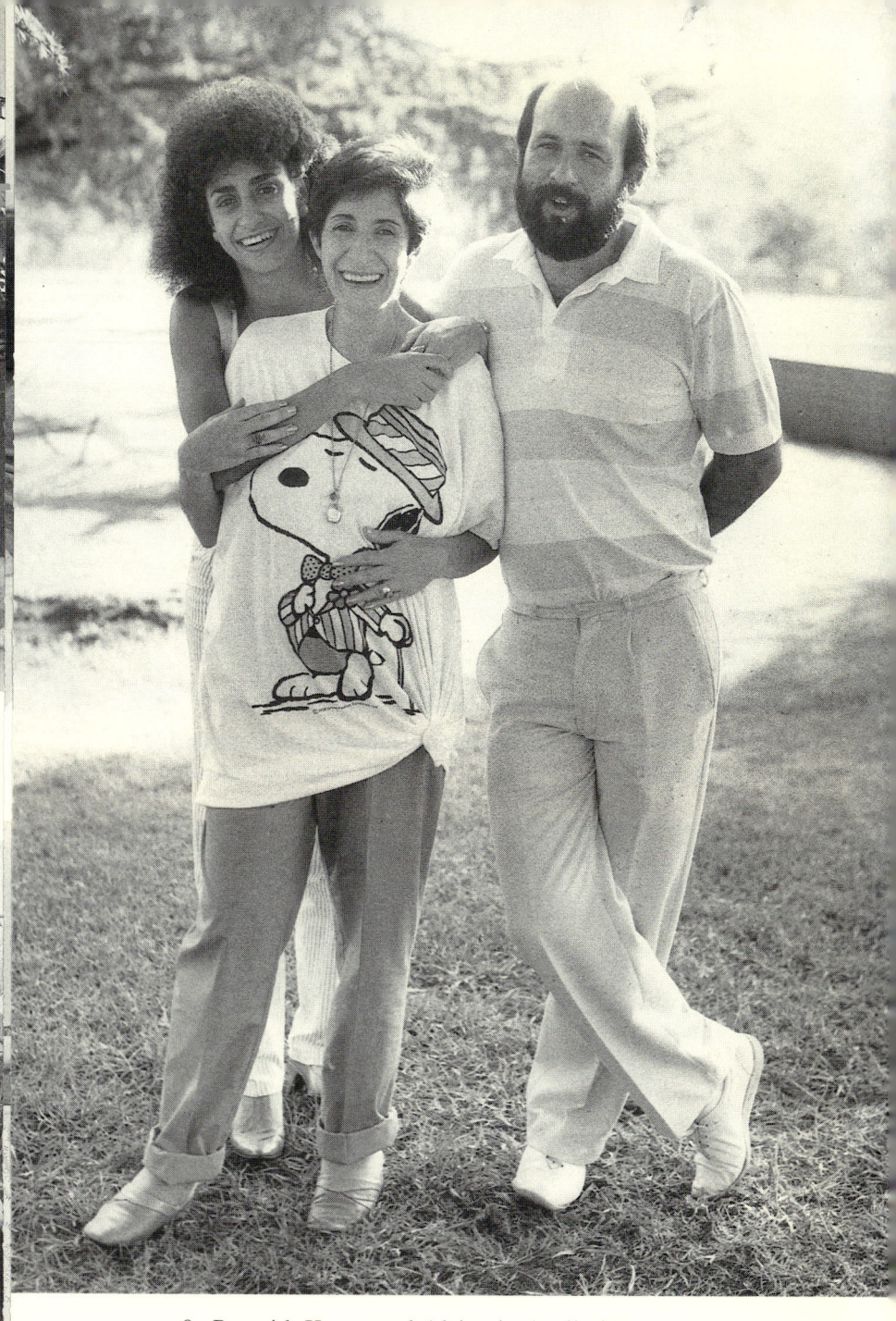

9. Pat with Karen and Alcino in April 1987.

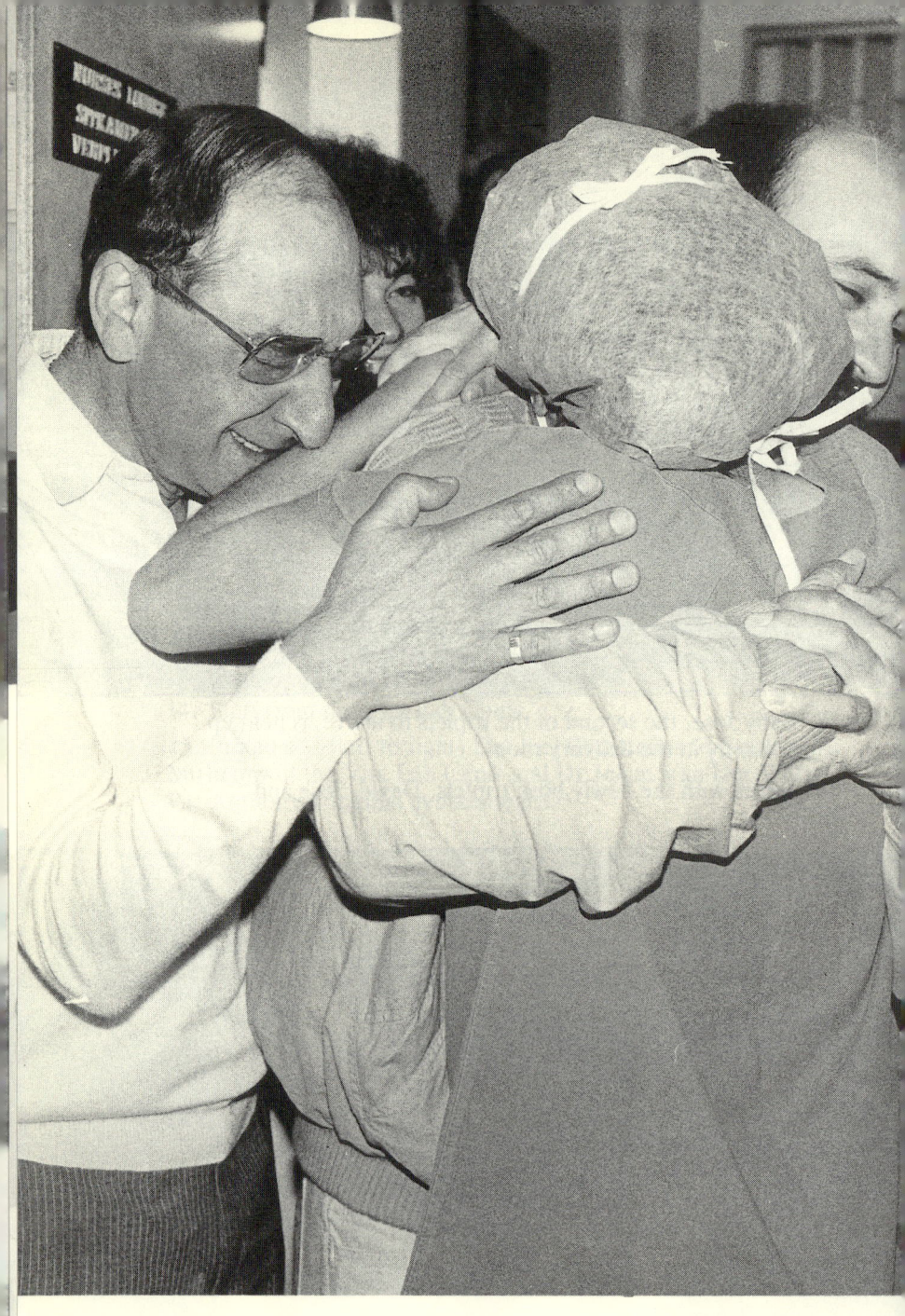

20. Karen, Alcino and Raymond in an emotional embrace outside the delivery room.

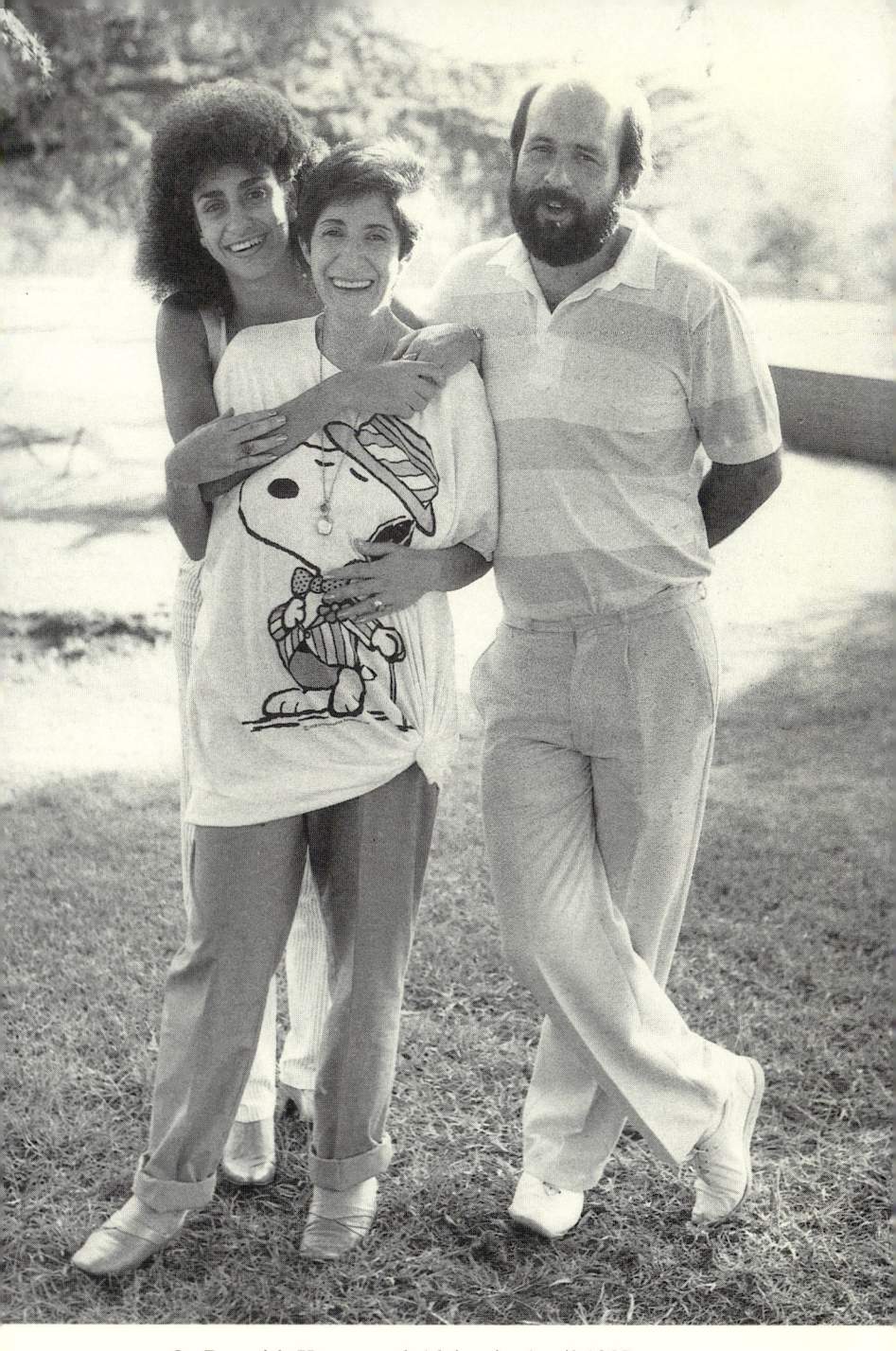

9. Pat with Karen and Alcino in April 1987.

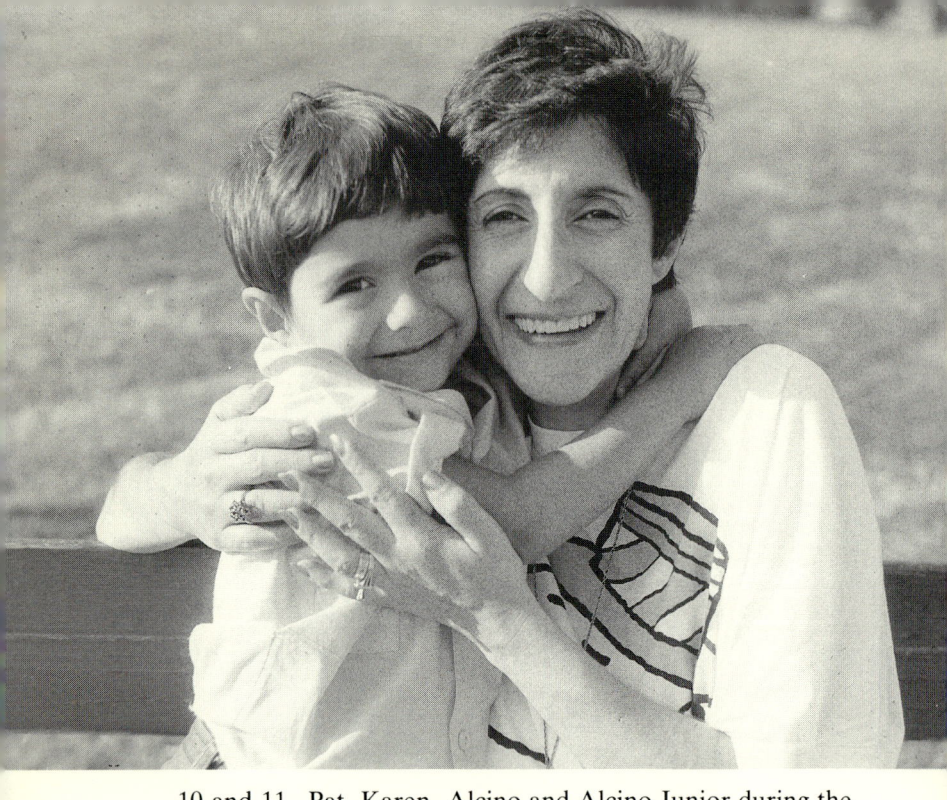

10 and 11. Pat, Karen, Alcino and Alcino Junior during the pregnancy.

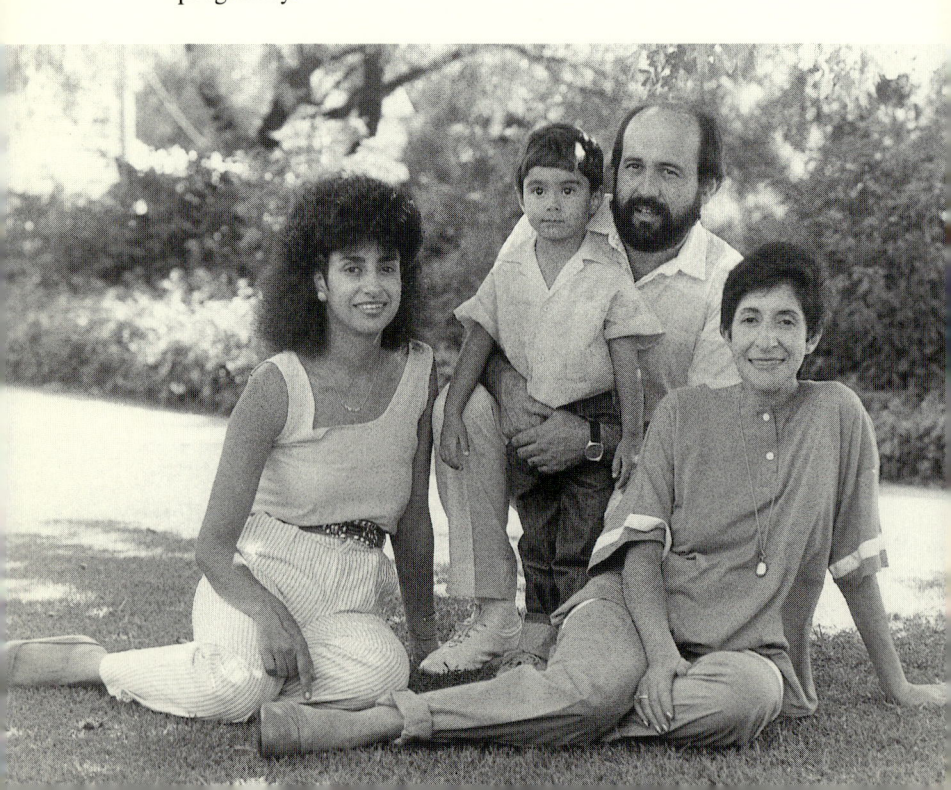

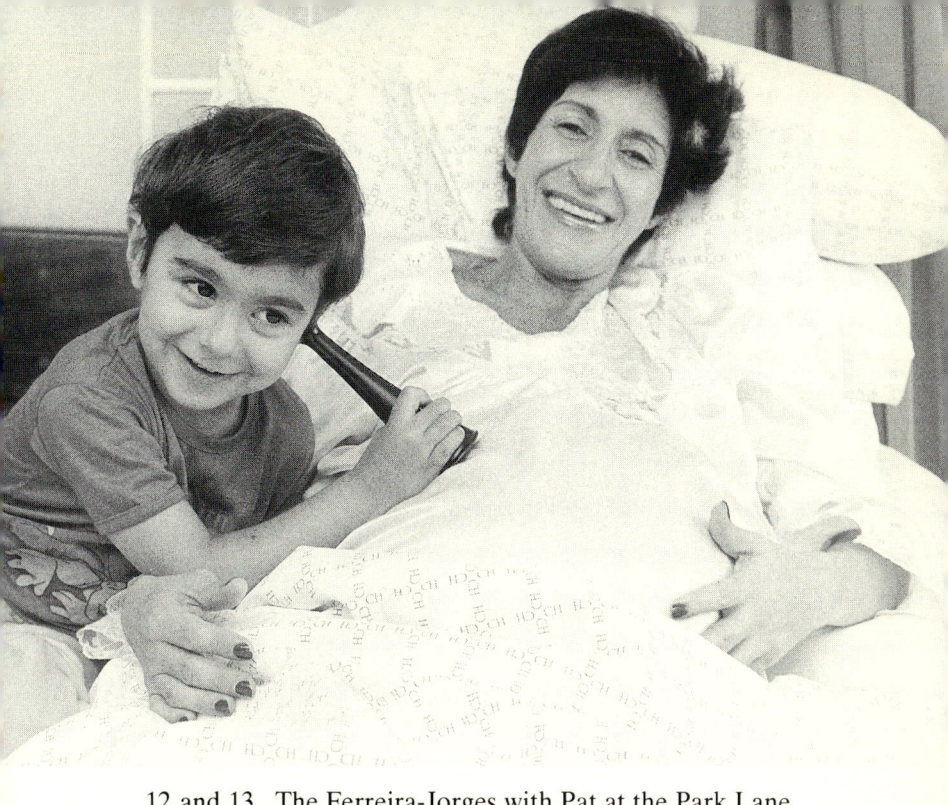

12 and 13. The Ferreira-Jorges with Pat at the Park Lane Clinic shortly before the birth.

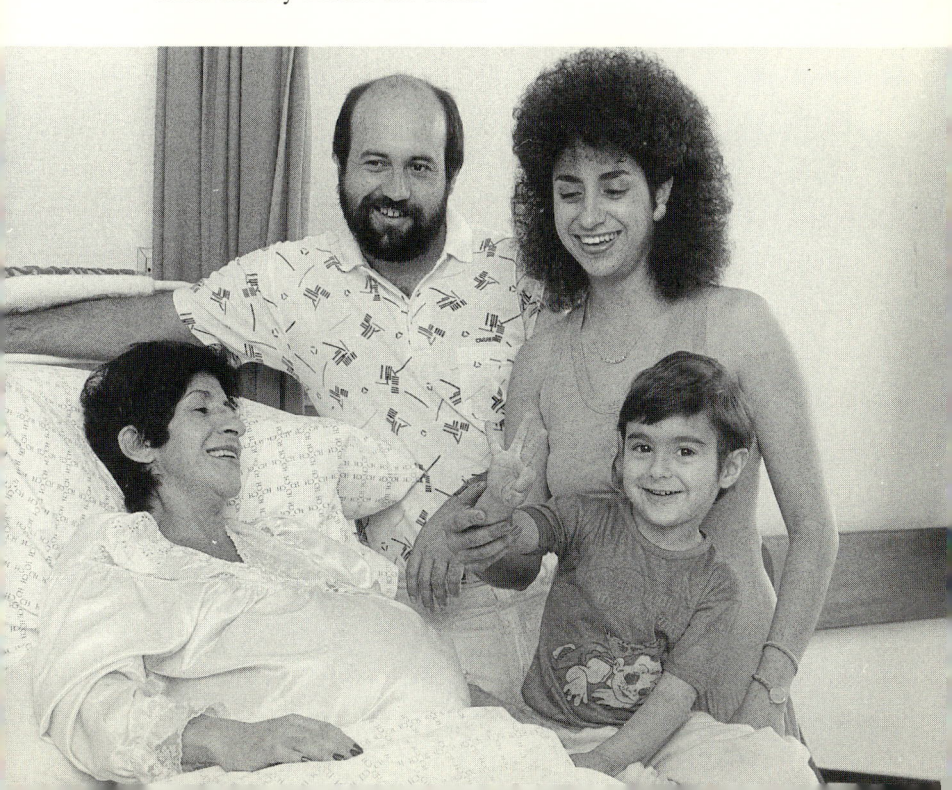

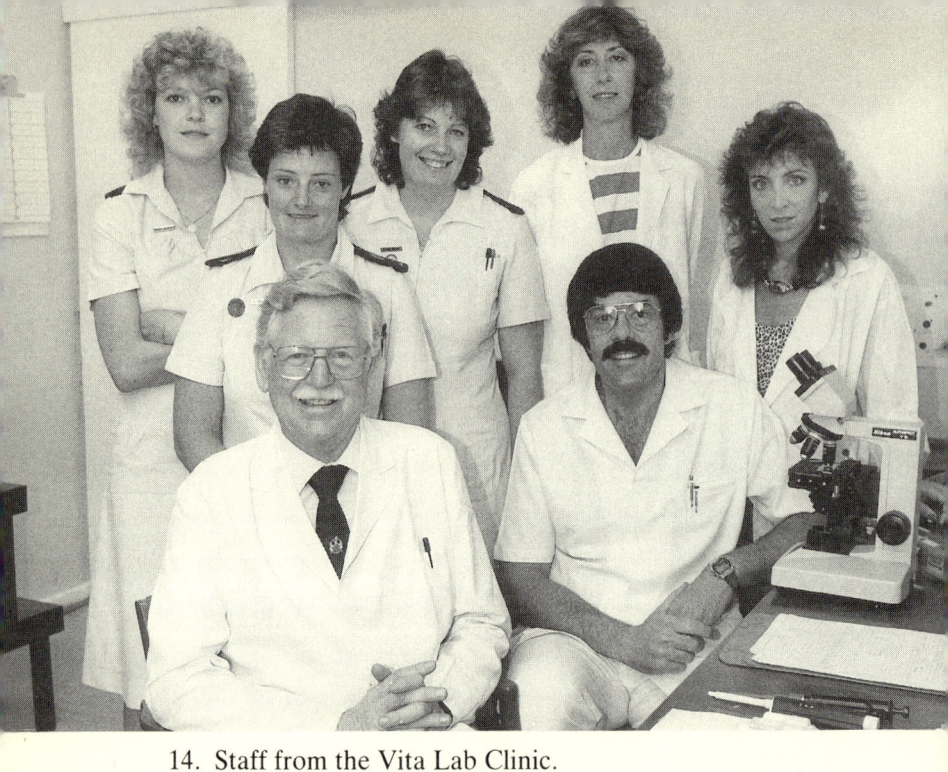

14. Staff from the Vita Lab Clinic.

15, 16 and 17. (left to right) Drs Joel Bernstein and Cecil Michelow of the Vita Lab Clinic and Dr Johan Van Der Wat, Pat Anthony's original gynaecologist.

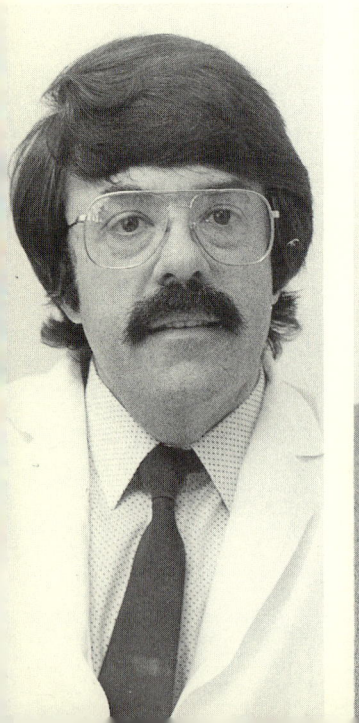

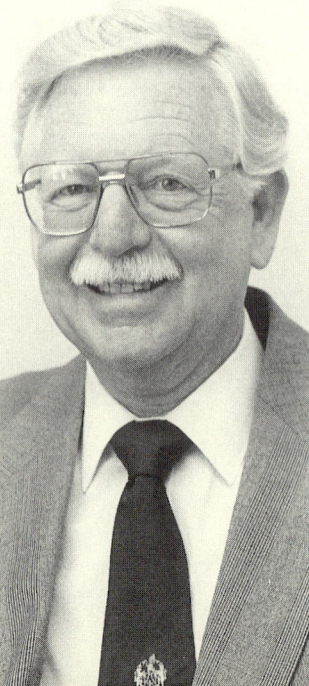

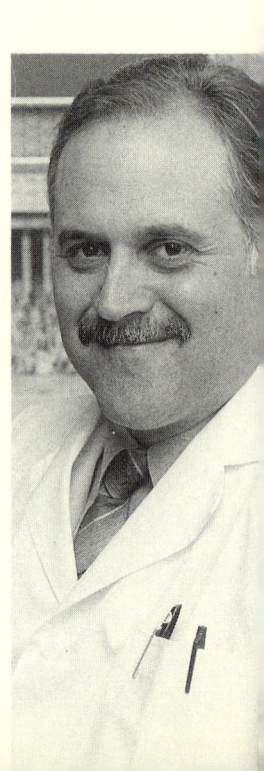

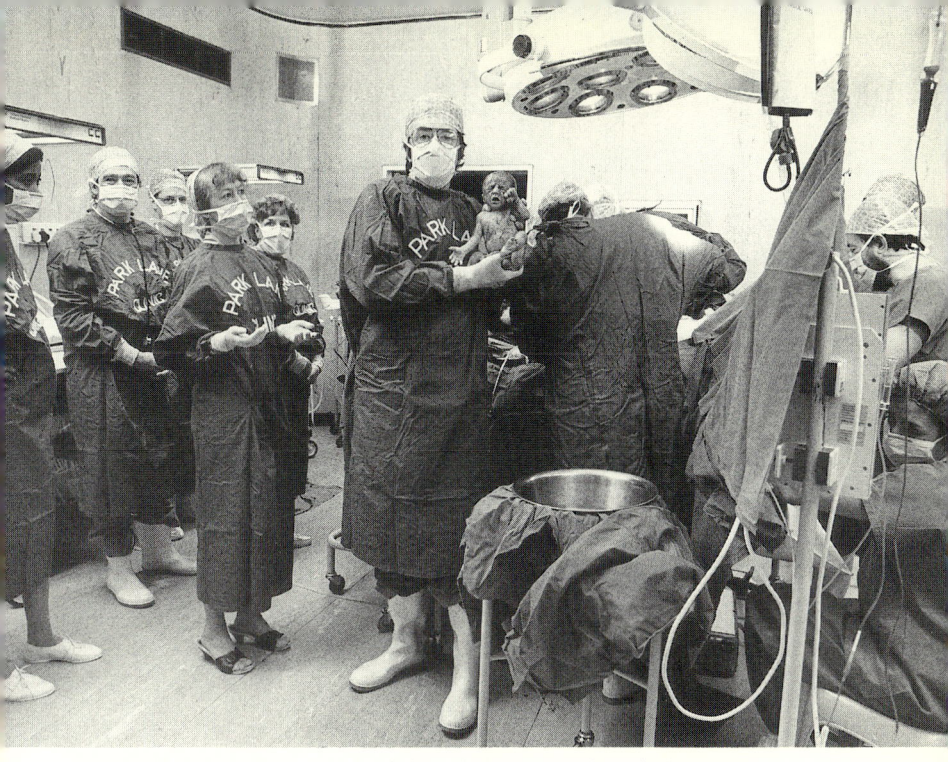

18. Baby Jose, the second of the triplets to arrive, is held up triumphantly in the delivery room.

19. Karen with the newly born triplets, David, Jose and Paula.

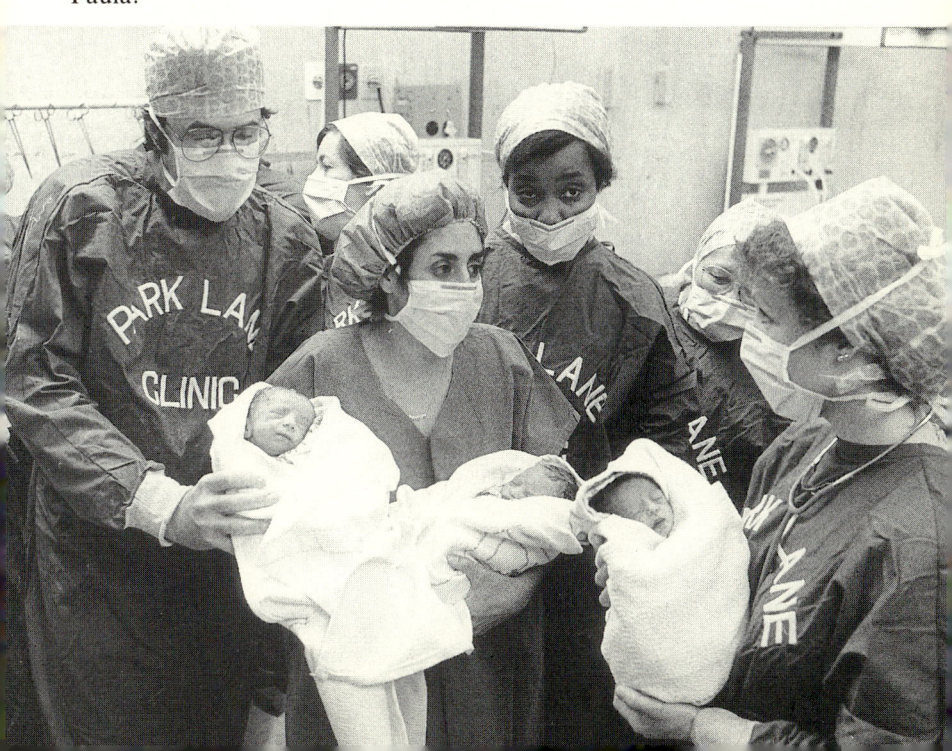

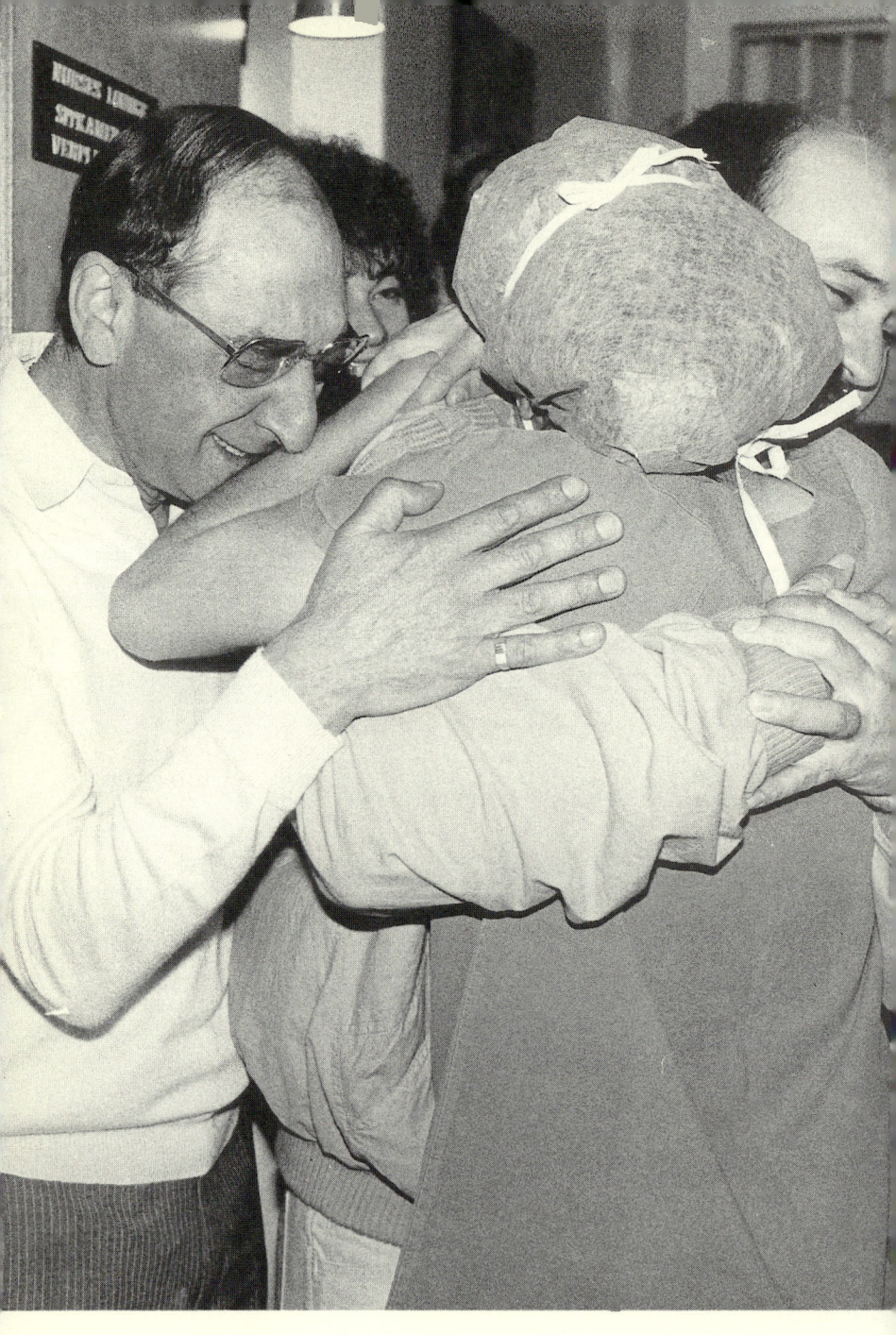

20. Karen, Alcino and Raymond in an emotional embrace outside the delivery room.

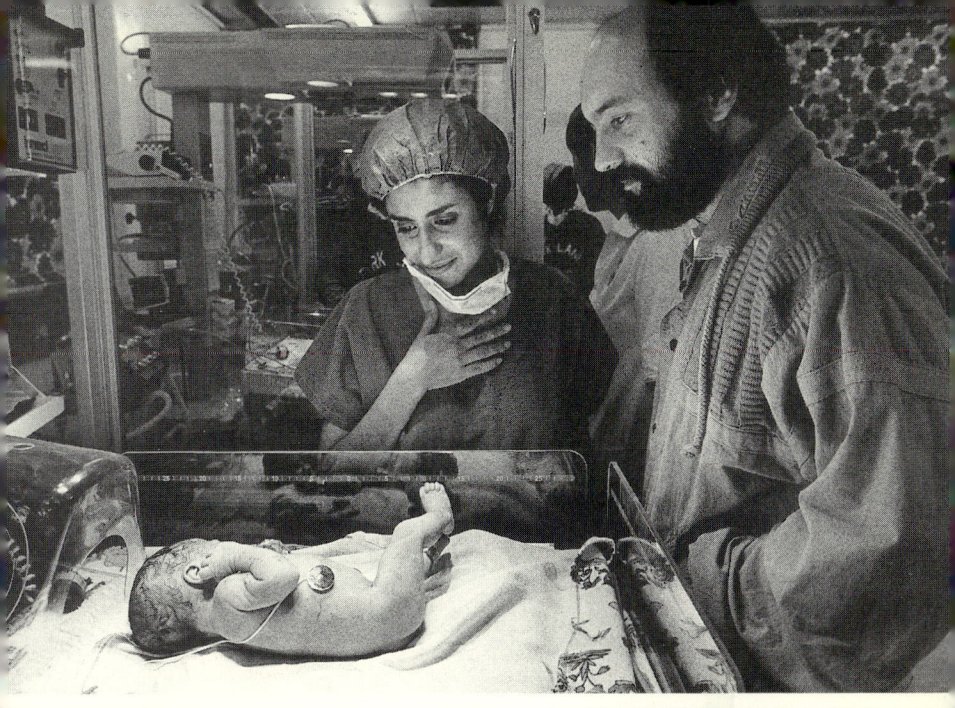

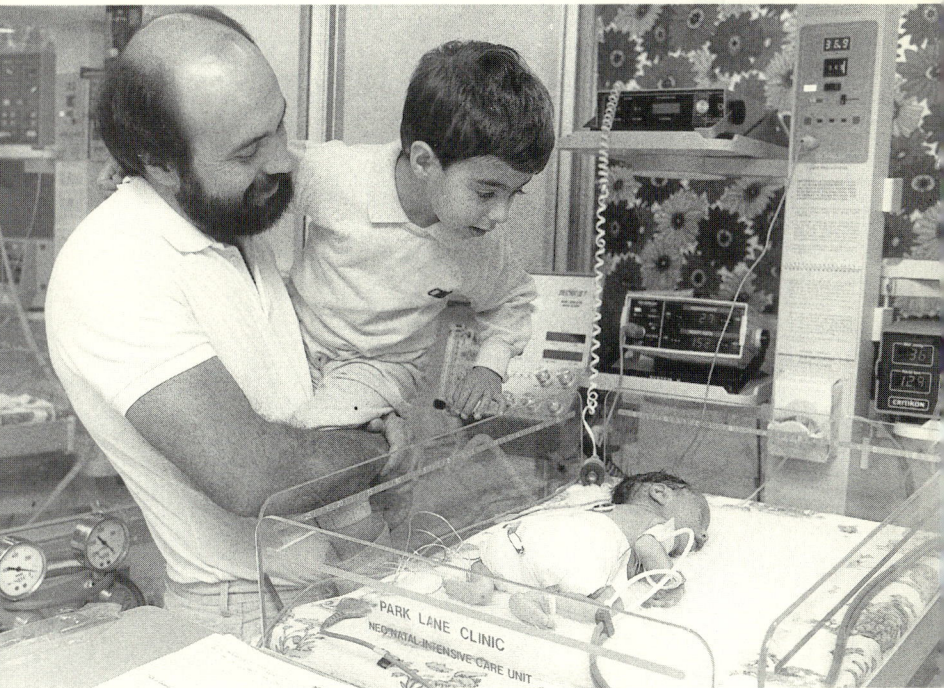

21. Karen and Alcino admire David, the first born of the triplets.

22. Alcino Junior meets one of the babies.

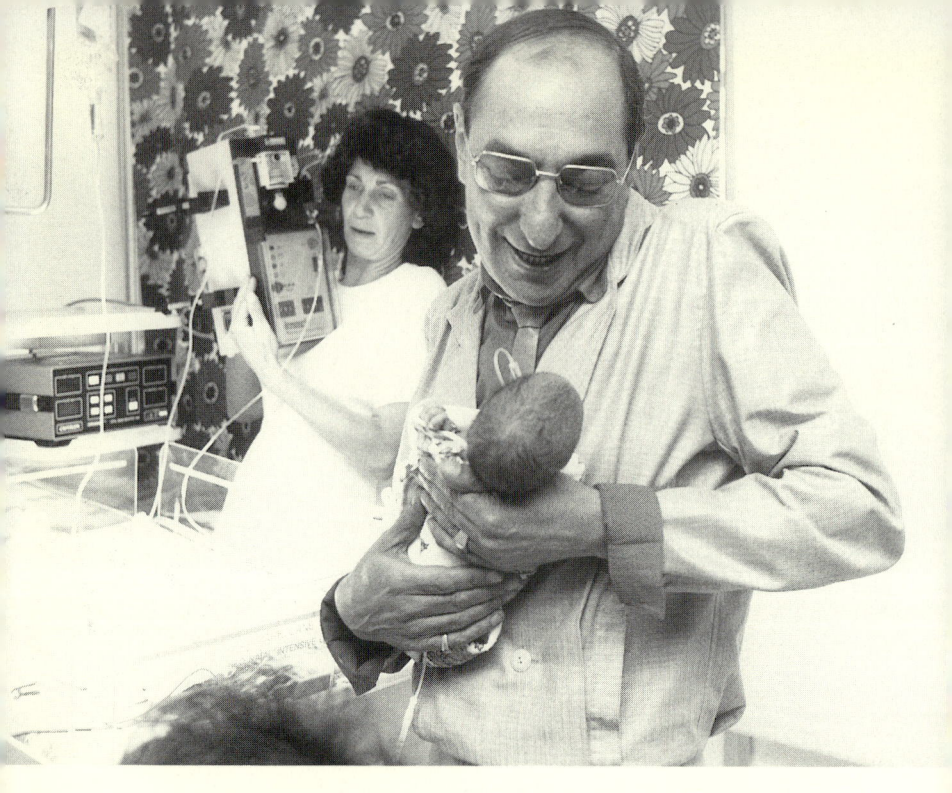

23 and 24. Raymond Anthony and his grandson Alcino Junior with the new members of their family.

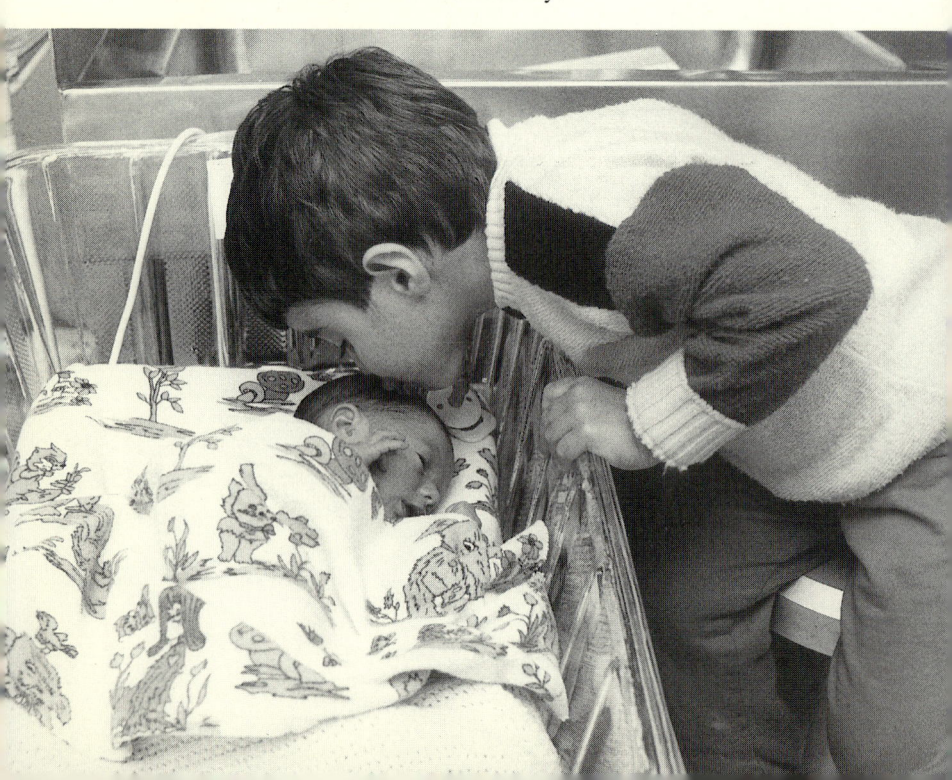

threatened to print a story if they did not co-operate. On the basis of a few questions answered by the couple, newspapers ran front-page stories without Joe or Magdelene's full consent. The publicity was out of their control.

'Don't let it just ride along,' Joe advised Alcino. 'Go public yourself in your own way, before the press find you. Then you will have a say in exactly what happens. You will control the publicity machine and you may be able to make some money to help the triplets.'

It was a crucial conversation, and one that Alcino related to his friend, British-educated avocado farmer, Howard Blight, a few days later. He was intrigued and wanted to help Alcino, whom he had patiently taught English after his arrival over the Angolan border more than a decade before. Howard, who had been sent by his prosperous father to Millfield, the famous co-educational public school in Somerset, and then to the Cirencester Agricultural College in Gloucestershire, was aware of international developments regarding surrogacy. The civil case over Baby M was being waged in the courts of New Jersey in the United States, and the Pope's condemnation of surrogacy had just been published.

'The time seemed right for the family's story,' he says. 'I thought it would show the acceptable side of surrogacy. It had a Catholic flavour, a South African flavour, and above all it was a story people, particularly women, everywhere would want to read.'

In Johannesburg the Vita Lab doctors, who were examining Pat every ten days, also warned her that the story could never be kept a complete secret. Although no one had yet told Pat, they realized they were dealing with a magnificent medical first. Not only was it the first time a grandmother had acted as a surrogate, it was the first time a mother had carried her daughter's children. And it was unique for a surrogate to have borne triplets successfully. It was also one of the first 'host' surrogacies where the babies would be the genetic children of both parents, using the surrogate mother's womb simply as an incubator.

Dr Michelow drew Pat to one side after a visit that March and warned her:

> Look, there is no way you are going to hide this pregnancy from your friends or anyone else. If you don't tell your friends about it then they are going to discover what is happening through the grapevine. Then they are not going to be friends any more, they are going to be upset that you didn't feel you could trust them. They are going to think you have been dishonest about the whole business.

Pat didn't take much notice. She was again living with her friends Mandy and Cliffie Jacob in their house at the end of the quiet Oakdene cul-de-sac. She waited and wondered what life would bring for the three babies inside her, did the bookeeping for the Tzaneen shop, and at night watched films on the television or played endless games of cards with Mandy, Cliffie and their three children. It was an odd existence for this woman who had always been so active, so much the centre of the Tzaneen family. Before her pregnancy, friends in Tzaneen would joke that they had never seen Pat Anthony walk down the street, only run. She was active and vital, but now she had to rest for the sake of the babies.

In her small room on the ground floor of Mandy and Cliffie's home, Pat had a small crucifix and she would pray silently that all would be well. And she remained certain of one thing. Her story must not be told to the outside world.

But during that March, as she continued to visit the clinic, Dr Michelow would ask Pat gently if she had reconsidered the publicity side of things. 'The world is going to want to see, they're not just going to want to read about it,' he insisted. 'They are going to want to look at you, to see what your face looks like. They will want to see pictures of the babies too as well as Karen.'

Raymond remembers the pressure on Pat.

We didn't realize the sensation of the story, and at one stage I think the doctor mentioned that it was quite a big breakthrough. He even mentioned certain figures that could be earned from newspapers and when Alcino and I discussed this at his place one evening we were adamant that we were not prepared to go into the limelight. In Johannesburg Pat felt exactly the same.

But after Alcino's supper party with the Darvases Raymond was persuaded. 'Because I saw that if we didn't do something about breaking it, then somebody else was going to do it for us. I suddenly knew it was going to be big and that we could raise money to put into trust for the triplets and Alcino, which we have now done.'

By the end of March there was only Pat who needed convincing. And finally, after a series of long-distance phone calls from Tzaneen, she was persuaded to go public for the sake of the triplets growing inside her. And Howard Blight, the avocado farmer who had been asked to contact a newspaper on the family's behalf, acted fast.

Because of his time in England he knew about London's Fleet Street, and described it to Alcino as 'the greatest hub of international news in the English-speaking world'. He believed if he took the story of a surrogate grandmother bearing her own grandchildren to a national newspaper there, the family would get a fair hearing. 'The story would be told without bias.'

On 1 April, just three days after the family's decision to go public, he picked up the telephone in the office of his farm in the hills outside Tzaneen and made an international call. It was 6.15 p.m. in London when the red phone of *The Mail on Sunday* news desk started buzzing and deputy news editor Graeme Gourlay picked it up.

The South African voice on the other end said, 'I have a story which involves triplets and a surrogate mother who has a very unusual relationship with the biological mother'. Then Blight, more unsure of himself than he sounded, started under Gourlay's questioning to unravel the full tale. But he was adamant that until a contract with the family was signed, giving money to the triplets' trust, no names could be given, no identities revealed.

However the reaction at *The Mail on Sunday* office was positive. Within 24 hours photographer Lynn Hilton, lawyer Christopher Cousins and myself, as features editor, were on a flight from London to Johannesburg, ready to take a light aircraft from Jan Smuts airport up to tiny Tzaneen. By the Saturday morning, 60 hours after the Blight telephone call, *The Mail on Sunday* had received exclusive pictures and words on the world's first surrogate grandmother.

As Pat, Alcino and Karen went into hiding in a suite of rooms at a Johannesburg international hotel, again it was Raymond who had to answer the questions. Within hours of *The Mail on Sunday* being distributed at 8.30 on that Saturday evening, 4 April, he was telephoned at his flat from every corner of the globe. Journalists from America, Japan, Australia, Germany and South Africa wanted the extraordinary story too. But Raymond would only say, 'No comment', two words that were to remain on his lips for most of 1987.

After a week, while the South African press led the search for the family and the Johannesburg *Star* bewailed the fact that it had been scooped by *The Mail on Sunday* under a headline 'They Caught Us Nappying', Pat returned to the Oakdene house.

Already she couldn't sleep flat on her bed, but only with pillows behind her so she could sit upright and breathe. Already her ankles were swelling if she stood for too long, or tried to cook a Lebanese dish for the Jacob family. Back home in Tzaneen, meanwhile, after the world-wide publicity, life was nearly normal, with Alcino going to his work every day and Karen running her exercise classes and tending three-year-old Alcino Junior.

But for Pat it was different. The grandmother at the centre of this remarkable surrogacy story was the target for most of the press interest, which never really faded away for the next six months. She could not go out to the shops and on one occasion she went so far as to wear a wig to the Park Lane Clinic, in case she was recognized. At Mandy and Cliffie's house she would never answer the telephone in case a journalist had discovered her hideaway.

Every day she spoke to Raymond and Karen, telling her daughter of every advance in the babies' growth. And then sitting upright in bed on 2 July, at two in the morning, Pat felt one of the grandchildren kick.

> I knew life was there for the first time and wrote down the date immediately. The next day I phoned Karen to tell her, you know. We were both very excited. It was fabulous. For the first time I felt the babies were a reality.

Chapter 6

When twins Danielle and Carla were born at the Queen's Medical Centre in Nottingham, England, it was a significant day not only for their delighted mother and father but for the whole future of artificial reproduction.

As these two babies were brought into the world on 6 November 1987, a meeting of doctors in London was debating whether children like them should be created at all. The Voluntary Licensing Authority, which lays down guidelines for the British work on *in-vitro* fertilization, argued at that meeting that eggs donated by one woman to a barren relative or friend could cause a 'tangle of potentially explosive relationships' in the future.

Danielle and Carla are the children of Ann and Steve Johnson, but they were only able to have the twins because eggs were donated by Ann's sister, Sandra (see above). Her eggs were fertilized with Steve's sperm and then implanted into Ann, who three years earlier at the age of 27 had been told she was going through a premature menopause.

The twins, although carried for 40 weeks by Ann, are genetically the offspring of their father Steve and their aunt, Sandra. While Ann plans to tell the children as soon as they can understand who gave the eggs and how they were conceived, the Voluntary Licensing Authority believes donors like Sandra should remain anonymous even if they come from within a close-knit family. Then, reasons the Authority, there can be no identity crisis in adolescence for children like Danielle and Carla; no questions later about exactly who is their own mother.

This is one of the latest ethical dilemmas to confront doctors pioneering new methods of conception, and one that our adult society can only struggle to sort out at the moment. None of the babies born courtesy of egg donation — and there are growing numbers — are old enough yet to put their own point of view.

In this ethical minefield, doctors, psychologists and sociologists are also trying to decide what the babies born through artificial insemination by donor (known as DI or AID), where the father plays no genetic role in their make up and sperm is given by another man, should be told when they grow up. And, more controversially, there are now also the children who have been carried by a surrogate mother, whose own egg has been used to conceive them, often as part of a commercial deal, to consider.

There is no doubt that artificial reproduction has brought a new dimension to family life and inevitably altered the whole structure of our society. Alexina McWhinnie, a senior lecturer in social work at the Buckinghamshire College of Higher Education in England, has warned that while test-tube babies will bring untold joy to their families they may also bring an entirely new kind of anguish and unthought-of divisions in the future. Rearing children where one genetic parent is quite absent from the home does not mean that his or her presence off-stage will not be felt in that family.

A teenager who knows that his genetic mother is his aunt may want to spend time with her, may wish to call his cousins his brothers and sisters or reject his 'nurturing' mother altogether. If the egg donor is a complete outsider then this young man or woman may embark on a search for the genetic mother in the same way as many adopted children now seek out their true parents. Who knows if Baby Cotton, the girl born to Kim Cotton, Britain's first commercial surrogate mother, will not in 15 years' time simply turn up on the doorstep of her natural mother's home after looking up the address in the London telephone book? If this girl is not told that she is indeed the celebrated Baby Cotton, who can say that she will not stumble across the truth as she goes through life? One slip of the tongue by a teacher, relative or neighbour is all that it needs.

To find any pointers to the future feelings of these remarkable children, we can only look at what has happened in the families where babies have been adopted, or conceived by the more traditional DI method.

Studies of adopted children show they often need to know where they come from and have an idea of what their natural parents looked like, did with their lives and why they were given away. The Swedish Committee on Artificial Insemination, which has recommended openness about genetic origins, has disclosed that: 'Research shows adopted children whose origins are kept a secret frequently know or suspect they are adopted, not because of any direct verbal communication, but through all the other clues which happen in any family.' A stray remark or the innuendo of a relative, or the embarrassment of a parent at a simple question from a child are enough to put the adopted boy or girl on the scent.

Although there are few reports of an adult needing psychiatric help as a result of finding out they are a DI creation, Alexina McWhinnie points out that there are family casualties: the mother who cannot bear the child conceived with the sperm of an anonymous donor to be in the same room as her husband; the wife who quarrels over the child and finally remarks, 'He's not your son anyway'; the child who suffers an injury and is taken into care and then adopted because the family can no longer accept him. There is even a case of a couple who moved to another country and postponed going home to visit their family for six years because their DI child did not have genetic characteristics which matched their own.

More alarming are the incidences of DI babies where the

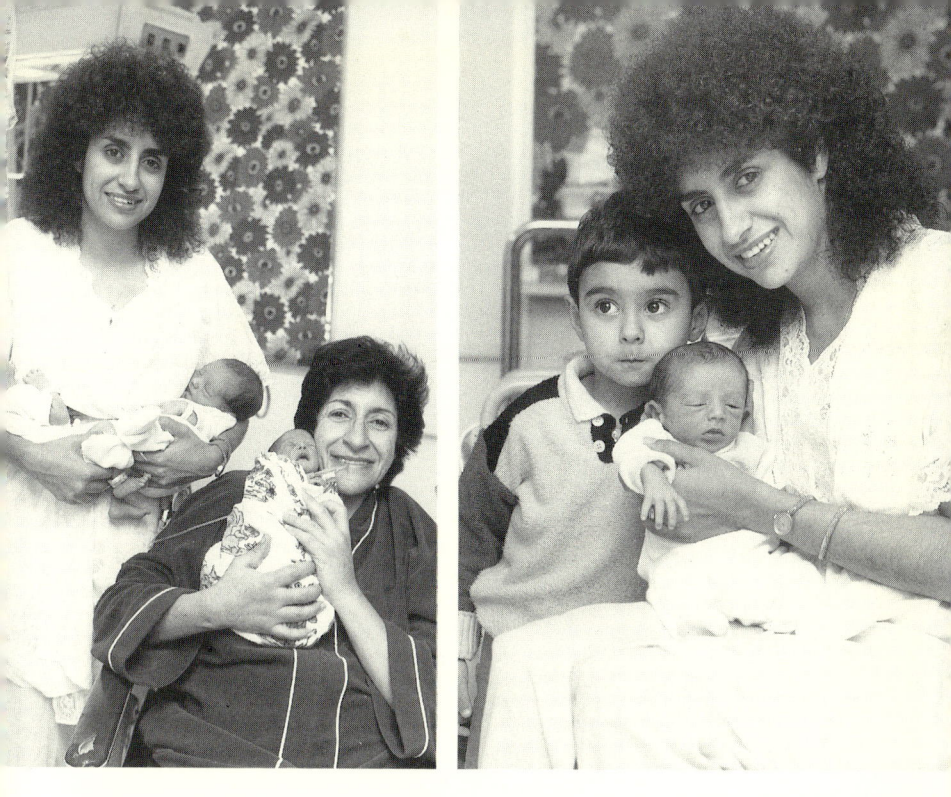

25, 26 and 27. Pat and the Ferreira-Jorges getting to know the triplets during the first few days after the birth.

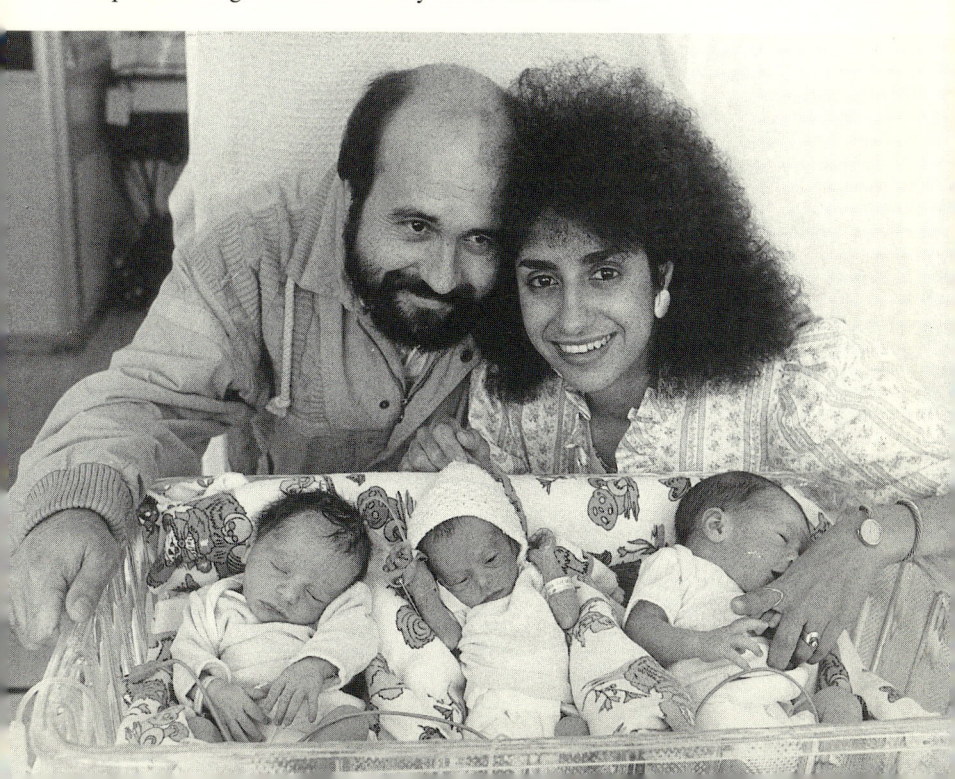

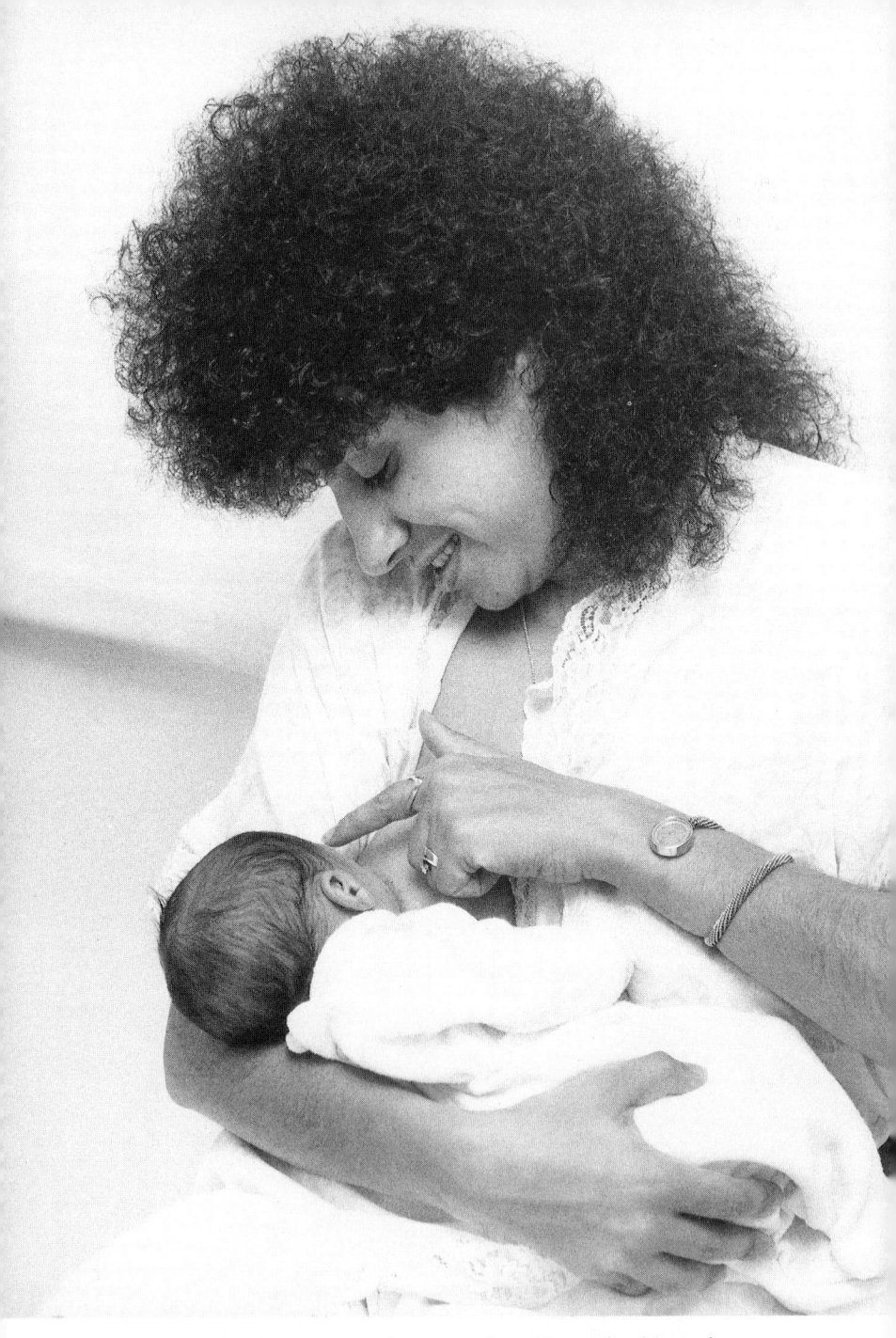

28. Following weeks of preparation, Karen is able to breast-feed her babies.

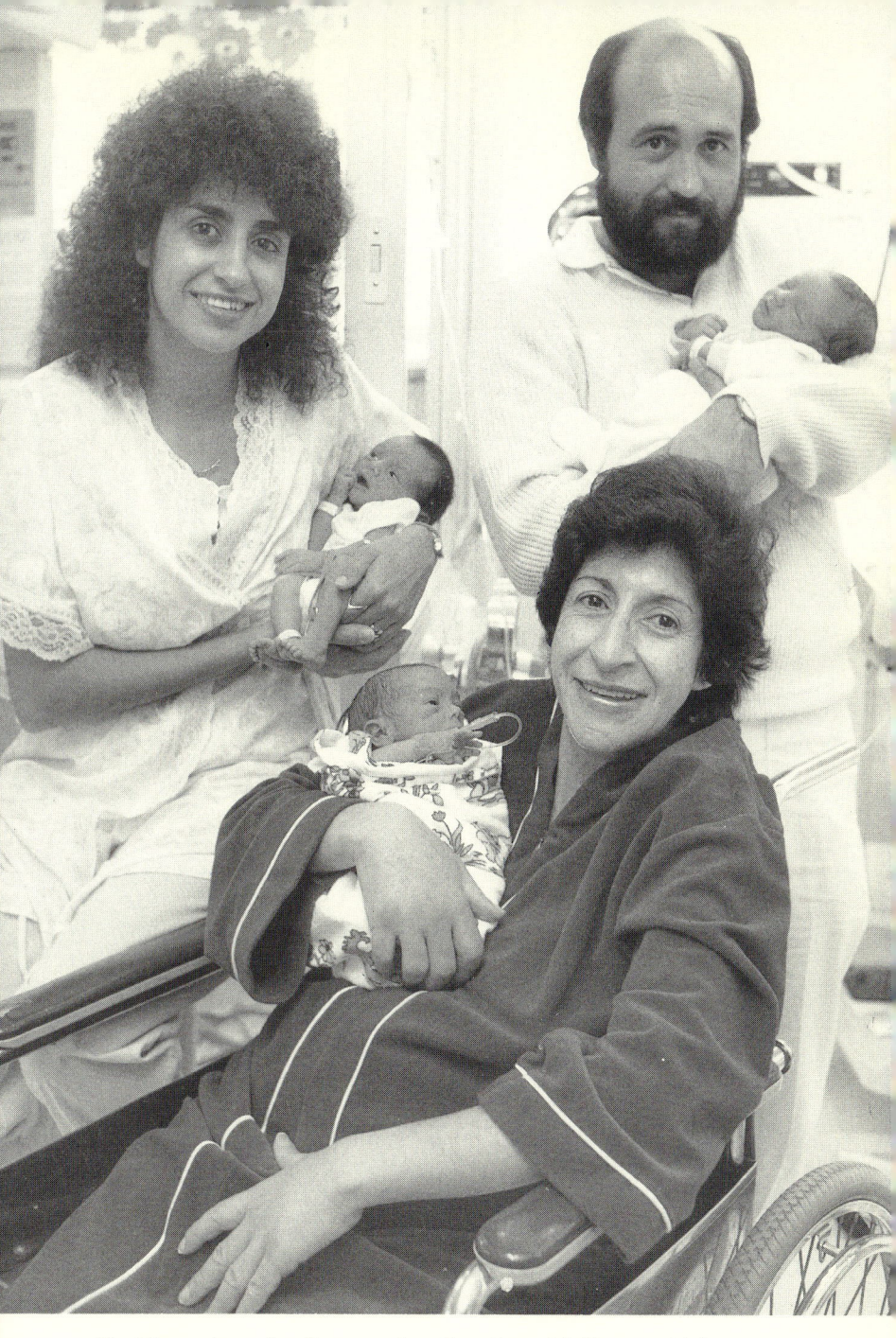

29. The unique family: grandmother Pat with Karen, Alcino and the triplets.

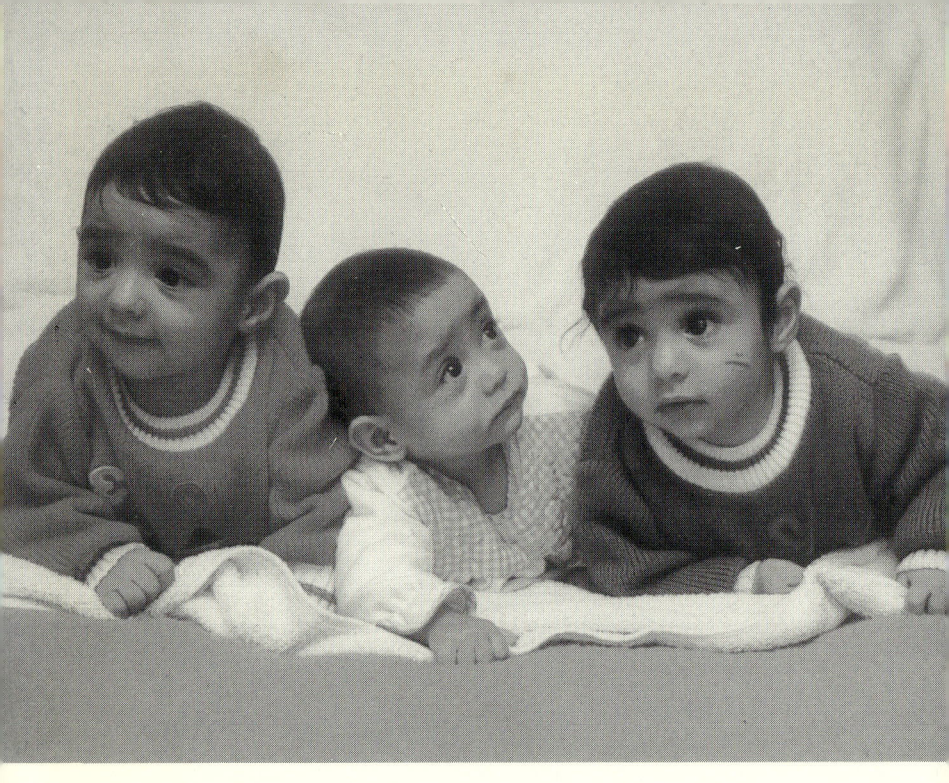

30 and 31. Seven months on: Karen, Alcino and Pat with Alcino Junior, David, Jose and Paula during a trip to England in May 1988.

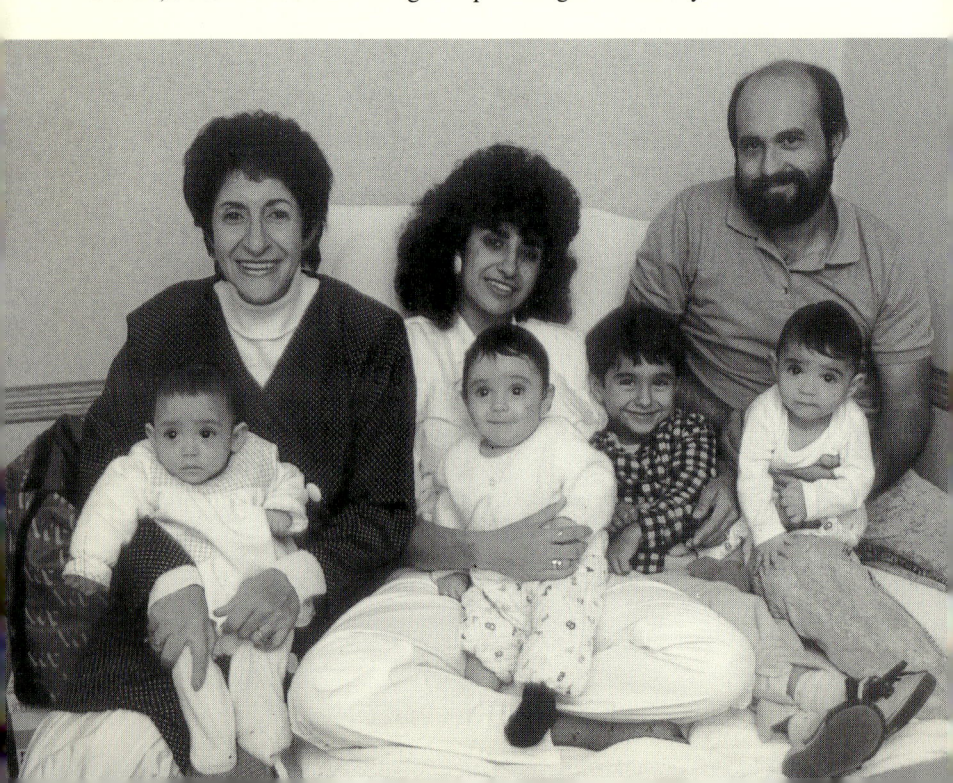

donor father is of a different ethnic background from what was stated and the DI adults who constantly search medical school records and year photographs for the student who fathered them, hoping to come across their true parentage.

Dame Mary Warnock, who headed the 1984 committee on *in-vitro* fertilization which laid down some ground rules in Britain, recommended that DI children should be given the information about their racial origin, and more importantly, their genetic health. There are many social workers who believe this does not go far enough. It is a half-way house where outsiders decide a young adult can have so much information about himself, but no more.

But to show how controversial the issues are, and how far away even the experts are from agreement, one only has to look at what the Voluntary Licensing Authority said about egg donations by relatives in May 1987. Then a leading infertility clinic, the Wellington Humana Hospital in London, clashed with the Authority over egg donations within the family and what the resulting children should be told.

Specialists at the Wellington Humana were given four months to change the practice of using donated eggs from relatives or, said the VLA, its clinic would be in danger of losing the Authority's approval. Three women at the hospital had just had babies as the result of eggs donated by their sisters. But the Authority warned that such close relationships could cause misery if the children grew up to discover their real background.

A spokesman for the Authority insisted: 'Egg donation should remain anonymous because the welfare and future happiness of the child is of paramount importance.' The hospital and its infertility team, headed by Professor Ian Craft and Mr Peter Brinsden, responded that they had tried to operate within the Authority's guidelines and in the best interests of their patients. Said Mr Brinsden, 'I see nothing wrong with egg donation from relatives. It is a compassionate attempt to solve infertility.'

Certainly the Australians, who have been front-runners

in test-tube conception and egg donation, agree with the British Authority. In 1982 the Ethics Committee of the Queen Victoria Medical Centre there approved the donation of eggs, only providing that the donor was anonymous and that the sperm of the husband was used to fertilize the donated egg.

But the intense ethical debate also covers the treatment of the tiny embryos created now in the laboratories of the modern western world, and even stored by freezing for use at some date in the future. For if we care about the destiny of the children born by egg donation, test-tube technology, DI or surrogacy, then what about those who are unborn? What rights should these pinpricks of human life be given by our society?

There are those, pro-lifers and feminist groups among them, who believe the human embryo has the absolute right to survival from the moment of conception or fertilization. That is when life starts. But English common and statute law states that the human child has no rights until it is born alive.

Test-tube baby pioneer Dr Robert Edwards claimed back in 1982 that it was ethical to use 'spare' embryos for clinical research and even to create them specifically for this purpose. He stated that embryos should be cultured up to at least 14 days if necessary, but there should be rules laid down about the length of time they could be frozen in embryo banks.

The whole debate has grown more controversial since the birth of test-tube twins to Mary Wright in Britain as described on page 35. Baby number one, created from a frozen embryo, was born 18 months before the arrival of baby number two, again the product of an embryo which had been unfrozen and implanted.

The case highlighted many unanswered questions. And it raised the whole issue of how long embryos, particularly if they are regarded morally as human entities, should be stored in laboratory freezers. The father of a frozen embryo may die before the pinprick of life is implanted and on its way to becoming a fully fledged human being. Should doctors then destroy the embryo because every child is entitled to two parents? The parents of frozen embryos may decide they no longer want the children they had prepared for. Should these embryos be given some sort of protection? Are the parents the people who order their destruction or the doctors at the clinic? If the unimplanted embryo is no more than a piece of property then presumably it can be disposed of by its owner as the owner sees fit? And what if the embryo is simply abandoned? Who decides on its future then?

The need for guidelines about frozen embryos was highlighted in Australia when a wealthy couple died in a car crash. They left behind them not a family but frozen embryos in a hospital deep-freeze. Lawyers were given the task of finding out if these human embryos had any claim on their dead parents' estate and whether they should be allowed to survive or simply be destroyed. In the end it was decided the embryos must be thrown away, that they did not have full human rights.

If the issue of freezing of embryos is set aside, then there are still tricky problems to overcome. When an *in-vitro* fertilization takes place many embryos are simply discarded. When Karen Ferreira-Jorge produced 11 eggs all of them were fertilized by Alcino's sperm and nurtured over 48 hours to become embryos. Four of these embryos were implanted in Pat Anthony, and the rest were thrown away. Could this process be seen as a mini-abortion, 'the destruction of a child being capable of being born alive', punishable certainly in Britain with life imprisonment under the Infant Life (Preservation) Act of 1929?

Such is the complexity of test-tube baby-making today. The first serious attempt in Britain to get to grips with the problems surrounding *in-vitro* fertilization, surrogacy, egg donation and the treatment of human embryos came with the Warnock Committee report of 18 July 1984, which followed two years of research and investigation into methods of helping infertile couples.

The Committee of Enquiry into Human Fertilization and Embryology made 60 recommendations. The main ones were that *in-vitro* fertilization, egg and embryo donation and artificial insemination were all acceptable as infertility treatments.

But the Committee insisted that research on human embryos should only be permitted under strict licence up to 14 days after fertilization, and a new independent statutory body must be established to control infertility services and to license and monitor closely all research in this field.

Significantly the Committee, which had been asked by the Conservative Government to examine the social and ethical implications of the fast-moving developments in test-tube technology and surrogacy, said there should be legislation to make surrogacy through either agencies or individual doctors a criminal offence.

It would then become unlawful to assist in the arrangement of surrogate pregnancies, whether for profit or not, and newspapers or magazines would be liable for prosecution if they carried advertisements for mothers or couples seeking a child. But a mother who was hired or a couple seeking a baby could not face legal retribution.

Two members of the prestigious Committee, Dr Wendy Greengross and Dr David Davies, were to disassociate themselves from the surrogacy recommendations. And while the bulk of the committee members thought it both distasteful and morally questionable for a woman to be willing to carry a child which was genetically her own and give it away to a father she had possibly never met, Dr Greengross and Dr Davies argued differently.

The two doctors agreed that money-making commercial surrogate agencies should be outlawed, but insisted that surrogacy could be beneficial on rare occasions to certain couples as a last resort. A non profit-making service might be a preferable option to unsuitable private surrogacy arrangements which could become the norm if surrogacy was banned outright.

At the centre of the whole debate was the question of

whether it is possible for a surrogate mother to carry a baby and be unaffected emotionally during or after her pregnancy. Does the bonding between a mother and her child happen in the womb or when the baby is first breast-fed and cuddled? Does the offspring of a surrogate mother become scarred emotionally when it is rejected, although it may have no memory of this event?

Now, four years on from the publication of the Warnock Committee's report, that debate is still going on. Surrogate mothers who have spoken about their babies illustrate the diversity of views.

In May 1986 in the United States Mary Beth Whitehead gave birth to a baby girl, now known in anonymous legal parlance as Baby M. She and Mary Beth were to become the central figures in the world's most controversial custody battle following a surrogacy pact.

Mary Beth at 29 was a devout Roman Catholic when she answered a newspaper advertisement appealing for surrogate mothers. This suburban housewife insisted to her husband, Richard, that she wanted to help infertile women because her own sister was unable to conceive and she had watched her misery.

The couple Mary Beth was put in touch with were biochemist William Stern and his wife, Elizabeth, a 41-year-old children's doctor. Mrs Stern was not infertile but did not wish to go ahead with a pregnancy because she was suffering from a mild form of multiple sclerosis.

Mary Beth was artificially inseminated with William Stern's sperm, went through the pregnancy without complaint and then, without any complications, gave birth to the baby. But during the delivery she changed her mind. 'I felt a lot of pain during the birth and at that moment I decided to keep her,' she explained simply afterwards.

Her determination was increased when her own family arrived in the maternity wing of the hospital and told Mary Beth that the new baby she was about to give away was a look alike of her 11-year-old daughter Tuesday. 'I thought I would be giving away a child to the Sterns but I never promised them my own daughter. The Sterns never even came to visit the baby until six hours after the birth.'

Because important papers had not been signed relating to custody, the baby – which even then Mary Beth insisted on calling Sara while the Sterns referred to her as Melissa – was not allowed to leave the hospital. Highly controversially, during those three days Mary Beth was allowed to breast-feed the baby, perhaps sparking off or strengthening the biological bond between daughter and natural mother.

Certainly Mary Beth was always to argue that the baby she had borne was rightfully her own. In the initial legal battle that ensued the Sterns were given custody of Baby M but when Mary Beth appealed to the American Supreme Court she was allowed to visit the child for two hours a week at a New Jersey State juvenile centre.

'My first visit there was the worst moment of my life,' she was to say later. 'The courts ruled that I was not allowed to breast-feed Sara, although I had when she was first born. I held my baby in my arms and she clawed at me, searching for my breast. I started crying and so did she. I will never forgive them for making my baby cry.'

Mary Beth has claimed that Baby M recognizes her as the natural mother and that there is a strong biological bond between her and her daughter. Whether this was formed in the womb or later because she was permitted to breast-feed and cuddle the baby no one knows.

But other surrogate mothers have felt entirely differently. Kim Cotton, for example, Britain's first commercial surrogate mother, insists: 'I have no regrets about making my decision.'

Three months after she gave birth Kim explained: 'At the end of the day I have the joy of knowing that out there in the world somewhere there is a couple who have the baby they longed for and that I have changed their lives. It still gives me a buzz to think about it.'

She went on to add that although in the hospital she had counted up the hours since the baby was born and taken away from her, this feeling evaporated when the child was given to her new parents and taken home. 'Then I could think she had her own mother looking after her and she was home and dry. Everything is in perspective for me now. I rarely wonder about her these days. But I'm sure I will always remember her birth date.'

Even when the child was nearly three years old Kim, who was never told the identity of the couple involved, was able to say in an interview with *The Times* of London that she had no interest in finding out about the whereabouts or the progress of the child she had once carried. (27 November 1987)

Following the publication of the Warnock Report and the Baby Cotton controversy, the government decided that, while a full debate on all the findings would take place at a later date, recommendations outlawing commercial surrogates would be implemented in a special bill as soon as possible.

Norman Fowler, Social Services Secretary, told the House of Commons: 'The case of Baby Cotton demonstrated the difficulties which commercial surrogacy arrangements can cause and the widespread public concern about them . . . I hope that the House will agree that action of this kind is justified and urgent.' The Surrogacy Arrangements Bill was published on 29 May 1985, and became the law that summer.

While babies born courtesy of modern medicine undoubtedly bring joy they present us with a moral nightmare. After the birth of the triplets to Pat Anthony, an article appeared in London's *Daily Mail* which summed up many people's fears about the future.

A.N. Wilson, celebrated commentator on modern Britain, wrote:

> Those of us blessed with children who have been born normally, and with comparative absence of complication, possess the greatest treasure, and the greatest source of happiness which there is.

Our observable happiness in our children must make the agony of childless couples all the more acute.

As it happened, the Ferreira-Jorges already had one baby. But as Roman Catholics they had been looking forward to a large family. Despite their Church's condemnation of these gynaecological experiments, were they not entitled to take advantage of modern science and possess themselves of that most innocent and delightful thing, a family?

It would be a hard man who said 'No' to this question. And yet it is difficult cases such as this which allow developments in medical science which are not necessarily in the general interest and which are not necessarily moral.

Those of us who aren't involved emotionally in the case should take a careful look at the implications of that granny giving birth to her daughter's triplets.

First of all, let us be realistic. It begins with a sob story, but how will it be used in the future?

Just as the busy working woman can now pay for someone else to clean her house, cook her meals, and design her garden, she will now be able to pay someone else to bear her babies in the womb.

A short visit to the doctor, and she will be able to leave a sufficient number of ova to be fertilized by the man of her choice. The resultant foetus, created in laboratory conditions, can then be implanted in the womb of granny or the cleaning-woman, or anyone else who happens to be available.

This is not merely aesthetically revolting. It is a denial, in human terms, of what motherhood is. The bonding which exists between a mother and her children must be intimately connected with the fact that, for nine months, she has borne them in the womb.

In the cases where children are not brought up by their natural mothers, there are doubtless all kinds of compensations. But what we are discussing in this instance is the near-certainty that women will want to use this method of birth simply because they can't be bothered to go through the turmoils of pregnancy and labour.

It is motherhood without tears. And that, like sex without tears, is a contradiction in terms. Tears and motherhood are essential partners, just as tears are an essential part of any kind of love.

You can see the way it will go. A film actress who does not want to spoil the shape of her breasts. A successful commodity broker who can't afford to have morning sickness when she should be on the line to Japan or Los Angeles. The model who does not want to have stretch marks or go nine months without high fees. Such women will be tempted to put their children through the test-tube and surrogate experience for the most trivial and selfish reasons. And God knows – literally, God only knows – the effect on these children of being born in this way.

Probably the answer is that if the children so born have a loving upbringing by parents who care for them they will be no worse off than children born in a normal fashion.

That may be so. But the idea of mothers opting for this method of birth for the most trivial of reasons is really the least of our worries.

Let's not forget that this method of birth was developed for cattle farmers. The idea is that if you have a sufficiently good combination of egg and seed it can be multiplied almost indefinitely.

Never mind triplets. It is technically possible, as with a herd of prize cattle, to produce a thousand-fold repetition of some winning combination.

The fact that this experiment has been successfully conducted in South Africa inevitably gives rise to Orwellian fears that it could be politically abused.

Hitler's doctors after all dreamed of achieving such a thing as this. And it would now be technically possible for the white embryos of what parents to be implanted in 10,000 black South African women.

For the duration of their pregnancies, it would stop them having babies of their own. And it would compel them to endure the burden and difficulty of pregnancy on the white parents' behalf.

Indeed such baby-farming could be used to multiply the white race to give them numerical superiority.

Now that is fantasy. But it is only political fantasy, not science-fiction. The truly fantastical thing — the ability of doctors successfully to implant someone else's embryos to grow to birth in another woman's womb — has already happened. It's science-fact, and we must now live with the consequences.

There is no such thing as a scientific invention which never gets used. If it is of use, someone will use it. We cannot un-invent this extraordinary thing any more than we can un-invent the nuclear bomb.

Nevertheless, we can urge the medical profession to proceed with caution. It is one thing to be able to do this thing. It is quite another to consider making it generally available in all cases of childlessness.

I find myself in the rather extraordinary position of being in wholehearted agreement with the Dutch Reformed Church, which has condemned the operation as 'meddling with God's business'.

The Catholic Church, likewise, into which these triplets will be baptized, has condemned the experiment as 'contrary to the dignity of the procreation of the human person'.

What is meant by that, I think, is that these experiments are treating the people who are brought into being in the laboratories as mere commodities. That is not how it appears in the present case to the triplets' doting parents, but it is how it appears in implications for the future.

You want a house? You go to the building society. You want a car? You ring up your Volvo showroom. You want a baby? Send for the specimen-trays and ring up the 'little woman' who was once frightfully good about producing twins for the Joneses.

But parenthood isn't like that. It is a mystery and a privilege. It is attended by luck. Parents, until yesterday, knew that they only had children because they were tremendously lucky. By removing that element of luck, I suspect that the South African doctors have done something sinister, and possibly evil.

Not everyone will share the controversial view of A.N. Wilson. Nor should they. But his article gives an insight into what the partnership between science and babymaking may bring to our society.

Chapter 7

At 1.20 on Sunday, 30 August, Pat Anthony was admitted quietly to the Park Lane Clinic, in a wheelchair borrowed from the hospital and carrying a brown and red walking stick which she had come to rely on for the few steps she could now make alone. The heavy weight of the three babies thriving inside her was beginning to tell. Her small ankles were now visibly swollen and she was tired out with the strain of carrying the extra burden inside her body.

Although it was still six weeks before the triplets were due to be born, the doctors had advised her to come to hospital for complete bed rest. Privately they believed that the triplets could be produced any day, premature like the majority of multiple births throughout history. But they kept these thoughts to themselves.

Pat herself was relieved to be at the clinic because now, into the eighth month of her pregnancy, she was feeling exhausted. Even the effort of getting up in the mornings from the single bed in the ground-floor bedroom at Mandy Jacob's house was proving a gruelling chore. And the night before she was admitted to the clinic she had confessed to Raymond on the telephone that she wondered how long she could go on.

But as she was wheeled swiftly through the clinic's main entrance and into the large lift to be carried up to ward three, one of the Park Lane's two maternity wards, she had a smile for the Matron, Beverley Frieslich, who guided the chair. Once in room number five of the ward, which was to become her temporary home, she turned to the matron and explained that because of her desire for secrecy she wanted to be booked in under a pseudonym, Ann Magua. Ann was Pat's second Christian name, Magua the maiden name of her own mother.

Already articles were appearing in the Johannesburg newspapers about the impending birth. There was continual speculation in their columns about when the South African surrogate granny, as she had come to be known, would have the triplets for her daughter. And although none of the press realized that Sunday that Pat had actually entered hospital, she explained to Matron Frieslich that to capture the peace she so desired the false name was a necessity.

Matron Frieslich, a tall and imposing figure, entered into the spirit of the occasion. She had already briefed the nurses on ward three about this important patient and asked them to respect her confidentiality. She said, 'I felt it was better to let the nurses in on the secret and trust them. I knew that in this busy ward they would soon find out who was in room five anyway. I tried to get them on to our side.'

But as Pat was tucked into her hospital bed that Sunday afternoon, it marked the start of a tortuous month when the tempers of the hospital administrators, doctors and nurses became frayed to the very limit. Angry words were to be exchanged between the world's press and the hospital for its handling of the whole surrogate grandmother affair and doctors soon came to disagree about the treatment of the surrogacy case they hoped would make their names.

The nurses in ward three were later to struggle to keep intruders from the South African press away from room five. They learned to trust nobody as journalists arrived at the hospital posing as visitors to other pregnant women on the ward. Already on 30 August the fire-escape entrances had been padlocked to stop reporters trying a less conventional route of entry and a screen was placed inside Pat's room so that anyone who did put their head around the door would see nothing.

Pat insisted that only a short list of family and friends could telephone her. They, she said, must use a secret code word, 'Sasha', or not be connected to her room. It was a system that was to work well and during her long stay at the hospital she never received any unwanted calls from the press, who besieged the switchboard at the clinic day and night once they discovered Pat's whereabouts.

With the bizarre security arrangements out of the way, the nurses conducted a sound scan on Pat, a check to see if the babies were still alive and growing. Although Pat was not told so that afternoon or subsequently, that first hospital scan revealed that two of the babies' hearts were beating away faster than that of the remaining child. It was an early indication that they were both boys and the third a girl. It was to turn out to be a very accurate reading.

In the evening at visiting time Dr Michelow paid a call on his precious patient and made his first prediction about when the triplets would be born. He considered a Caesarian operation should happen any day, 3 September at the earliest. Pat's health was the paramount consideration, he said, and if she was under too much strain then the babies must be brought into the world prematurely.

Another visitor that night was Dr Van Der Wat, the doctor who had referred Pat to Michelow for treatment. The Afrikaans doctor was more cautious. 'Because there are three babies inside her they will all be smaller than normal. They are 33 weeks old but in size and development they will be like 30-week foetuses,' he warned.

The next morning Pat was seen by Dr Bernstein, the second member of the Vita Lab partnership. He disagreed with Michelow. 'We want her to go to the 24th of September,' he insisted. It was the first indication of a growing rift between the four doctors, a division that was to become more serious and create hideous tensions as the days wore on towards the end of Pat's pregnancy.

Although Pat and her family were totally unaware of it

then, the sparring amongst the Vita Lab trio of doctors already had a precedent. Michelow, Bernstein and Jacobson had all been partners in Vita Lab, the infertility clinic, when Pat had first visited the hospital the previous year. But now, because of deep disagreements over the workload share-out in the partnership, it was in the process of disintegrating in the most acrimonious atmosphere.

By the time Pat reached the last days of her confinement Bernstein and Jacobson, who wished Vita Lab to survive without Michelow, were barely on civil speaking terms with the older doctor. Michelow himself felt he was being squeezed out of the clinic he had played a significant role in founding.

The surrogate grandmother unwittingly became a catalyst for the developing rift. If the babies were born alive and healthy then the Vita Lab would become famous. It would be transformed from being a little-known laboratory with an unremarkable success rate to one that had achieved an incredible medical first. Now the three doctors really had something to squabble over.

This unhappy state of affairs manifested itself in outright verbal warfare over how Pat Anthony should be treated; if there should be a Caesarian operation at an early date, or whether she should be allowed to continue her pregnancy until the last possible minute. As the days went on, with Pat tucked away in room five of ward three, the whole hospital seemed to become unwittingly embroiled in this partnership rift.

Some of the nurses backed Michelow's theory that Pat's welfare must take precedence. He argued that premature babies of one kilo in weight could now survive with intensive care. Whatever happened nothing must jeopardize the life of Pat Anthony or else a medical first would become a medical disaster.

Other nurses, like the Scottish Matron Groat, a resilient and good-humoured spinster from the Shetland Islands who ran the labour ward with a rod of steel, supported Bernstein's view that as far as possible nature should be permitted to run its course. If Pat Anthony could carry the three babies nearly to term then so be it. 'They are still tiny, these babies,' she would caution Michelow crisply. 'Let's not rush it.'

When Pat had been in hospital for 24 hours the three doctors wheeled an ultra scan machine into her room and discovered that the smallest baby already weighed 1.6 kilograms, heavy enough to survive outside the womb if Pat went into labour. It was a relief to all of them. But pressures of another kind were just beginning to manifest themselves.

On Tuesday 2 September, when Pat had been at the clinic for only 48 hours, the Johannesburg *Star* carried a front-page story saying the South African surrogate granny had entered hospital on the Monday. The date was wrong but the story was accurate enough to spark off a renewed frenzy of press interest. *The Beeld*, an Afrikaans national newspaper, telephoned Raymond in Tzaneen pressing for details. He would only say no comment. At the hospital a photographer from the *Star* staged a continuous sit-in for the day in the entrance hall. But, to the family's amusement, the cameraman watched Karen Ferreira-Jorge walk through the lobby into the lift to visit her mother without recognizing her and lifting his Nikon to take a photograph.

From that day on Karen would take elaborate precautions when arriving at the hospital to make sure she was not recognized. She wore a headscarf and would come in through a side door at the back of the clinic. Driving home to Mandy Jacob's house, where she was now staying with Alcino Junior, she would take a tortuously long route to make certain no journalists followed her to the secret address.

But the South African press did not give up easily. A reporter from the Johannesburg *Sunday Times* was soon to discover Mandy working at her hairdresser's shop and accost her about 'your friend Pat Anthony who stays with you'. It was a redundant effort though. 'She is a distant cousin of my husband's,' lied Mandy, quaking inwardly. 'I don't really know Pat Anthony at all.' And the reporter, after hovering outside the shop, went away fooled by Mandy's denial.

At the hospital Pat would spend the days doing the accounts for the Tzaneen gift shop and reading an endless supply of paperback books. She would rarely get out of her bed apart from to bathe in the morning, using the tiny shower adjoining the private room. She chatted to her close friends on the telephone but was careful never to disclose more than the briefest of details about her general health. She wanted the possible date of the birth and everything intimately connected with her pregnancy to be kept out of the newspapers. And she knew that one anecdote unwittingly relayed by a friend to an outsider could mean she was back on the front pages and the pressure to find her would begin again.

During the long hours, punctuated only by hospital breakfast, lunch and dinner served by the nurses, she had time to brood over the remarkable venture she had started. There was no doubt in her own mind that she was doing the right thing for her daughter. But she was wise enough to question her own emotions. And in her diary, eight days after entering the hospital, she was to write:

> I still don't think these babies are mine and I don't think I ever will. I know that they are Karen's and Jorge's own babies. I just want to see them born well and healthy.
>
> When they kick I don't feel maternal, it just makes me laugh. I don't feel as though I am going to be a mother, only a grandmother. I am just the carrier, the incubator for my grandchildren.

The words were brave, for it was not as though Pat was a woman who had never known maternal stirrings. When Karen and then Colin were born she had experienced all the pangs of new motherhood, the need to nurture her young. But this time, reasoned the commonsense Pat, things were very different and had been from the start.

She was to attribute her rational attitude to the actual moment of the implant of Karen's eggs into her body in January. 'I was awake when the implant happened and it was very clinical and very technological. It helped me to realize that these children who would grow inside me were not mine and never could be,' explained Pat in the hospital.

'If I had been put to sleep during the implant then I would not have been aware of what really happened. With the doctors and nurses in their green gowns it was just an operation like any other. It sort of drummed it into me.'

But if Pat was perfectly in control, Karen suffered a short bout of nerves. She moved to a suite at the Sunnyside Hotel near the hospital, and had plenty of time to dwell on what life would be like when the babies actually arrived. 'I am excited about the date getting nearer,' she explained, 'but I am worried about what I will feel for them because I have not carried them. I have to start preparing myself now, making myself realize they will really be my sons or daughters.'

Although the Vita Lab doctors never voiced their fears to the family, they too were concerned about what exactly Pat and Karen would feel when the babies came into the world. They could not start to predict how the emotions of the two women might run as no surrogacy pact between a mother and her daughter had ever happened before. They were steering into uncharted waters and they knew it.

A resident psychologist with the Vita Lab was drafted on to the medical team to counsel Pat, Karen, Raymond and Alcino Senior, but it was a thankless task. Each one of this remarkable family seemed mentally prepared for what the future held. Pat herself would have little to do with the counselling and Karen was soon more interested in discovering the psychologist's thoughts on how Alcino Junior would react to three younger brothers or sisters, than how she would cope when the triplets were first placed in her arms.

Karen said, firmly:

I certainly don't feel any jealousy about my mother carrying my babies, I do miss being pregnant because that was something I enjoyed with Alcino. I used to sing and talk to him when he was in the womb. And I am certain that helped build up a relationship. But surrogacy does have its compensations. It has brought my mother and I even closer together. We talk about the babies together, and I can see them kicking now. I am really starting to believe they belong to me.

Pat was diplomacy itself. She was always careful to refer to the triplets as 'the babies' rather than 'my babies', not only in front of her daughter but in the hearing of the whole of the astounded medical team. Nurses on the ward who in the tense weeks running up to the birth predicted that Pat would have last-minute feelings of remorse about giving up the children growing inside her were to be proved wrong.

Even the experienced Matron Groat was to say privately that she believed Pat was enjoying the pregnancy and would have psychological problems when the children were born. 'She will get the baby blues like any other woman who has just given birth,' she predicted. 'She may feel very lonely once the triplets have been taken from her and given to her daughter.'

Yet as the coldest Johannesburg September anyone could remember went on, Pat showed none of the warning signs. Mentally, she was adamant that the birth would leave her unaffected. Physically, her blood pressure remained normal, her ankles became less bloated when she took water tablets, and only the relentless heartburn she had suffered through the whole pregnancy stayed with her night and day.

Karen began preparing in earnest to breast-feed the babies by taking hormone tablets and using a breast pump. She had practised breast-feeding on friends' babies in Tzaneen and although the progress was slow, by the middle of September she was producing ten mls a day, a feat in itself. Pat, sensible as usual, had decided she would take pills to suppress her milk supply and rejected the suggestion by Dr Bernstein that she should help feed her daughter's babies. 'They are not mine to feed anyway,' she argued gently.

But if all seemed calm on ward three of the Park Lane Clinic during that September, in the real world outside the surrogate granny was the subject of endless newspaper and television debate. The pressure was relentless, almost as if the South African media had no other story to tell. Yet it was only on the Sunday morning of 20 September that the Johannesburg *Sunday Times* was able accurately to pinpoint Pat's whereabouts within the clinic. They emblazoned this information on the newspaper's front page and said that Pat was booked into the hospital under the name of Magua.

The details, although innocuous in themselves, had been leaked by hospital staff to the newspaper and immediately jeopardized the babies. Although the article contained a fabricated piece of information, that Pat had a craving for ice cubes, it was near enough to the truth to show that a line of communication had been forged between the *Sunday Times* and a source right inside the hospital.

But before that Sunday morning was out Pat had been moved by nurses to room seven on ward three in a renewed effort to stop her room being invaded by journalists. Matron Groat, in charge of the clinic that day, was perturbed by the newspaper article. 'We have to ensure security for high-risk patients like this,' she insisted. 'I am worried that if a reporter just marched into Pat Anthony's room she could be shocked and go into labour before her time.'

Yet despite the press microscope on the hospital Pat's pregnancy continued smoothly. The only false alarm about her health had happened on 10 September when at 8.45 in the morning the doctors on their early round discovered that Pat's blood pressure had soared. Immediately the labour ward was booked for the following day and the medical team told to stand by. But by noon the blood pressure was back to normal and Dr Michelow called off the Caesarian planned for 11 September.

As the days dragged on the relationship between the three Vita Lab doctors worsened. Dr Michelow, who had first accepted Pat as a patient and potential surrogate mother, insisted he should be allowed to make the final decision about the birth date. But Bernstein and Jacobson, his partners who had also helped care for Pat since the year before, insisted they must also have a say in this extraordinary event.

Although Michelow had hoped that for Pat's sake the birth would happen sooner rather than later, by 16 September the pregnancy had reached a highly crucial stage, a stage that meant the Caesarian operation could not occur for another fortnight. Between the 35th and 37th week of pregnancy a baby's lungs are in a crucial state of development. At 34 weeks even a premature child of very low weight is more able to cope with life outside the womb than one of 35 or 36 weeks. At 37 weeks this danger period, which even doctors still do not yet fully understand, is over.

Dr Michelow explained:

> If anything happens to these babies and they are born disabled or even die then the fingers of the world will be pointed at us, the doctors. It will be a disastrous end to what should be a triumphant medical first. The family would be destroyed, too, if anything is allowed to go wrong.

So the waiting went on. It was agreed that if Pat's blood pressure rose during the next fortnight or she became too uncomfortable carrying the three babies then the birth must be arranged. If not, then the triplets would not be brought into the world until October.

It allowed more time for disagreements between the doctors to worsen. Now the constant pressure from the South African newspapers and television network, SABC, was beginning to tell on the medical team.

During that curious fortnight, despite the wishes of their patient Pat that there must be no publicity and her anonymity as far as possible should be preserved, Dr Michelow and Dr Van Der Wat were the target of intense lobbying to appear on SABC to talk about the surrogate grandmother.

SABC, and in particular the television station's woman producer Carol Charleywood, brought pressure to bear on the two doctors. There were ill-veiled threats that if the doctors did not appear then and there, their careers in South Africa might be jeopardized. And the two doctors were well aware that SABC is a government-run organization, often used as a mouthpiece for the Afrikaans-dominated National Party.

Finally, ignoring the requests of Pat Anthony, Dr Van Der Wat and Dr Michelow appeared on the Afrikaans programme, 'Network', on the evening of 20 September. The two doctors discussed the whole issue of ethics in surrogacy but also talked about how Pat had come to the Park Lane Clinic to make her plea about carrying her daughter's children a year before.

The normally good-willed Pat was outraged. Despite her immobility she decided to call a meeting of the four doctors and her family at her hospital bedside. It was a remarkable decision under the circumstances but Pat was determined that as the patient her wishes must be obeyed. Her case must not be intimately discussed in public.

In her room on the afternoon of 24 September she told the doctors she wanted an undertaking from them that details of her treatment should remain private. They must also agree that when the birth happened they must not speak to outsiders.

Bernstein and Jacobson, who had never sought publicity over their involvement in the case, accepted the diktat from Pat and her family. Dr Michelow was less willing to conform to the guidelines set down and standing by Pat Anthony's bed that afternoon he argued that the South African nation had a right to know about the surrogacy.

However the most determined to make the story public

was Dr Van Der Wat.
He said:

It is important to explain to the South African public what is going on. They are ignorant about surrogacy and what it entails. Unless the full facts are told then the government here will ban all future surrogacies. There will be pressure from ordinary people as well as government ministers and the Dutch Reformed Church to do so.

Yet Pat won the day. Sitting propped up with five pillows, more or less confined to her hospital bed, she persuaded the medical team to remain silent. She badgered them with the words, 'Do as I wish or don't come into the hospital theatre for the birth.' That was enough for her to get her own way. 'You are lucky that I haven't insisted on complete anonymity,' she said.

By now Pat, who like her daughter Karen believed the birth should be at the last minute and if possible not until 14 October, was beginning to feel the wear and tear of her pregnancy. On 25 September, a Friday night, she began to have contractions and was unable to step out of her bed unaided by nurses. Yet by the next morning the alarm was over. Anti-stress tests on the babies showed all was well and Pat decided to persevere for another few days.

It was only three days later, when a sonar scan of the triplets showed the smallest, lying on Pat's left-hand side, was not growing like the other two, that the doctors named the day.

They decided that on Thursday morning at six o'clock Pat Anthony should give birth to her daughter's children. The relief that finally a decision had been made was immense, but still Pat insisted that the hour and the day must be kept a secret. The theatre was booked by Matron Groat in the name of Magua and the three paediatricians from Johannesburg's Morningside Clinic, Doctors Maxwell Hopp, Mervyn Ossip and Rene Heitner, who would look after the babies from birth into their first few weeks, were told of the appointed time in the utmost confidence.

Pat, still determined that the birth should take place without a blaze of instant publicity, even turned away the auxiliary who came to prepare her for the operation 48 hours before. 'That can all be done later,' she protested.

On the night of 30 September she settled down to sleep at nine o'clock, her door closed to everyone apart from the night nurse from Euxton, Lancashire, who sat and listened in case she should call. The next day Pat Anthony hoped to achieve a miracle.

Chapter 8

The night of Wednesday 30 September was a tense, turbulent one for Karen and Alcino as they waited in the local hotel for the alarm clock to shrill at five in the morning, the signal for them to drive the few minutes to the Park Lane Clinic to see their children born. In the spacious suburbs of Parktown, surrounding the hospital, the doctors and nurses in their comfortable homes also lay awake waiting for dawn to come. For everyone it was going to be a momentous day, the conclusion of a medical experiment which had already shocked the world.

At 4.30, soon after daybreak, Pat began preparing herself for the Caesarian, with the help of night nurse Karin Peters. Still full of fun, Pat joked to the nurse that very soon the babies would not be her responsibility any more, but her daughter's. Although she would be awake throughout the operation, her body numbed with an epidural injection, she was not afraid.

She tidied her dark hair, applied her make-up and soon after 5 a.m. was wheeled calmly down the corridor of ward three to the Clinic's labour unit. Although it was early, new mothers were already feeding their babies in ward three. But the nurses, who had now developed an admiration for the surrogate grandmother, closed the doors of the rooms as the wheelchair slid past so no peeping eyes would recognize her and see that Pat Anthony had been moved.

In the labour ward Pat was left in a side-room to rest and wait for her family to come in to see her. Downstairs the hospital's night watchman prepared to let the four key doctors, Matron Groat, and a clutch of handpicked nurses into the hospital through a private door reserved for specialists and administrators.

This medical team of 11 would be present at the birth, and each one of these men and women had been sworn to total secrecy. So too had the paediatricians who would take charge of the treatment of the three new babies from the moment of their birth. They would stand by in the main theatre of labour ward number one and monitor the babies once they were born. Doctor Ossip would take care of the first to arrive, Dr Heitner the second, and Doctor Hopp the last of the experienced trio.

It had all the makings of a military operation, with Matron Groat in charge of the manoeuvres. Ideally the babies should be lifted from Pat's body in less than a minute. Everyone in the theatre, from Dr Michelow who would be making the first incision and performing the operation to the lowliest swab nurse, must know exactly what job they had to do, and when to do it. Never before had a surrogate mother given birth to triplets. No one in the theatre, despite their joint wealth of experience, could tell precisely what would happen.

At 5.30 Pat Anthony was taken into the theatre to be put on an epidural drip and the medical team started dressing in their masks and gowns. The excitement was obvious, an undercurrent running right through the team.

In an ante-room normally used by nurses to take refreshments, Raymond and Alcino sat and waited, Raymond chain-smoking his high-tar cigarettes. Karen was handed a green gown by Matron Groat and instructed how to put on her mask. She would be going into the theatre to watch her babies being born.

Through the open theatre door Pat could be seen lying quietly, her body starting to freeze from the chest down as the epidural began to work on her. She looked a small figure on the large operating table, tended only by the anaesthetist, Dr Colin Nates. But even in these last 30 minutes she had the strength and courage to open her eyes and call her son-in-law Alcino to the doorway.

Looking at Alcino, to whom she had always been so close, she waved and called out, almost in triumph, 'Very soon you will be a father again. You mustn't worry.' The remarkable gesture had Alcino searching for his handkerchief and wiping his dark eyes, overflowing with tears of gratitude towards his mother-in-law. 'I will be happy,' Pat said, 'if my daughter and you are happy.'

The moments ticked by towards the 6 a.m. deadline. Outside the hospital South Africans began to wake up and prepare for another ordinary working day. But in theatre one of Park Lane's labour ward events were far from ordinary.

Pat had asked for her face to be shielded with a small screen from her body so she would not see the babies arriving and taking their first breaths. Beside her, on the left-hand side, was a little footstool where Karen would sit throughout the birth. When the babies were born, Matron Groat and the doctors decided, Karen would then move away from her mother to the three incubators in the room where the triplets would be placed.

Beside each incubator stood one paediatrician, their task about to begin. At ten minutes to six Karen took her seat, chatting to her mother and holding her hand tightly. On Pat's right-hand side, on another neat footstool, was Dr Jacobson, ready to talk the surrogate grandmother through the birth, explaining precisely what was happening, calming any fears.

His presence was important, a gesture of care and concern for Pat's mental wellbeing during the operation when she would hear the first sounds made by the babies she had carried for so long, as they were taken from her body. She, and no one else in that room, could judge just what her reaction would be to the cries of her grandchildren. Would this courageous grandmother feel any maternal cravings as the babies were handed to her daughter, never to be her very own? Or would she just treat their first mewings as marking the moment she triumphed against all the medical odds?

Dr Michelow headed the medical team that day. Dr Van Der Wat stood by his side, charged with the task of deftly stitching Pat at the end of the Caesarian operation. Dr Bernstein would be handed the babies the second they were born, ready to act if anything was wrong. Then the nurses would carry the babies to the incubators and the waiting trio of paediatricians.

The operation began soon after 6 a.m. There was hardly a sound in the theatre, only the doctors murmuring instructions to each other and at the head of the theatre table Dr Jacobson and Karen could be overheard whispering to Pat. Yet the anticipation and nervousness could be felt right around the room.

The doctors bent their heads in their blue plastic caps over the numbed body of their extraordinary patient and forgot all the differences of the last weeks. Now the team of 14 was working together to make history and ensure that three perfect babies were the result of their year of effort. Very soon Dr Michelow turned to Karen and Pat to warn that the first baby was on its way. He had hold of a foot and the child, a baby boy, came out quickly. The time was 6.10 precisely and Karen remembers exactly how it happened.

> I heard a husky little cry and then this turned into a healthy bawling. Suddenly I had a son, David was with us. He was handed from one doctor to another and then away to the nurses and an incubator across the theatre. My mother smiled at me and it was obvious she was elated too. I didn't need to be told that my son was perfect. You could hear that.
>
> We waited for the second baby to be born. It was only one minute later but it seemed a long time to us. Then Jose came along, again crying lustily as he was lifted up by the doctors.

It was then that Pat murmured to her daughter that she hoped the third baby inside her body would be a girl. Although neither Karen nor Pat knew it, a scan two weeks earlier had confirmed that the smallest child was indeed a girl, but the doctors and nurses had complied with the family's request that the sexes of the three triplets should remain a close secret until the moment of birth. But it took another two minutes for the third child to draw its first breath, two minutes that seemed like an eternity for the doctors. Lying underneath the placenta was the little girl Karen had waited for for so long.

The doctors knew that this smaller third baby was in danger. If she was not brought into the world quickly she could stop breathing. And Dr Michelow and his colleagues were aware of something else that worried them greatly. Two days before the birth a scan had revealed that this baby, only four pounds in weight, was lagging behind her two brothers. She had stopped growing and if she had remained much longer in the womb would simply have faded away, starved of the nutrition she needed to put on weight. It was this knowledge that prompted the decision to go ahead with the birth on Thursday, 1 October.

Now, as the theatre rang with the cries of David and Jose, Dr Michelow battled to bring the little girl into the world. As he searched inside Pat for the baby, he discovered that the sac surrounding her had no water inside – a sign that she would not have survived for much longer. He felt a hand but could not find the baby's foot to lift her into life. Then at 6.14 there was a whimper and she had arrived, tiny but perfect. 'My mother and I were both crying when the doctors took her from my mother. I wanted her so much and this was the very last chance I would have to bear a daughter,' said Karen.

It was only then, with each of the three babies lying in their individual incubators, that Karen left her mother's side. One at a time, she stood by the five and a half-pound boy, then his four-pound brother and finally she admired her tiny baby girl — the girl she would call Paula. Beyond the theatre doors, Karen's husband Alcino waited. 'Karen came running to me in her theatre gown and mask,' he said in a voice choked with emotion,' and flung herself into my arms. She told me I had two boys and a girl, just what I had always hoped for.' Standing outside the theatre doors he had heard the cry of the first baby – David – then, a minute later came the wail of Jose. 'But I grew worried as I searched for the sound of a third baby and none came. It was only now that Karen was able to tell me that all was well and I had a daughter too.'

The three babies were checked by the paediatricians and pronounced healthy, then swathed in white they were handed one by one to Karen. It was an emotional moment, as the doctors and nurses stood by and watched. For although these newborns had not grown in her body, they nestled in her arms content to be loved and nurtured.

The moment the babies were born Pat was given a drug to make her sleep so that the sounds of the babies' continual crying around her would be dulled. She was not aware of Karen holding her children for the first time, or the exclamations of the joyous doctors declaring the babies whole and perfect.

As the triplets were put back in their incubators and wheeled away to the hospital's intensive care unit where they would spend their first few days, Dr Michelow said:

The birth went so successfully we did not even have to use extra blood. It all went better than our wildest dreams. Pat Anthony now has three marvellous grandchildren. Karen has three bonny babies. For a surrogate mother of 48 years old to have carried her daughter's three babies right until the 38th week is incredible. The screaming of the babies when they were born was unbelievably loud. It is rare you hear three newborn crying at the same time in the same operating threatre. It was just the sound we wanted to hear.

Dr Bernstein was ecstatic too:

As each baby was born I couldn't help but hold it closely. I just wanted to touch them because what had started life in a little white dish had actually become a human being. It's amazing, even for me as a doctor, to see something that in January was only a tiny speck, the size of a pinprick, could now be held in my arms. I am certain myself that what Pat Anthony has done for Karen is totally acceptable. There was no payment, no commercialism. What Pat did for her daughter was a pure act of love.

For Pat herself, left in the operating theatre to be checked by the doctors as her daughter and babies moved off in a triumphant cavalcade down the corridor, it was to be a few hours before she could voice her feelings. Raymond, always a devoted husband, admired his new grandchildren and then went into the theatre to sit with his wife.

And when Pat awoke later in her room he was to tell her, 'This is the greatest proof of a mother loving her daughter that the world has seen. We have had so much joy from Alcino Junior, and it was always sad to think he was the only one. You were the driving force behind this whole attempt to give him brothers and sisters.'

They were words which Pat needed to hear at this time, because although she was never to suffer any major postnatal depression or even the 'baby blues', she had after all undergone a major operation and was battered physically by the experience. Yet she never wavered in her belief that the babies were for her daughter. She insisted:

I will never claim them or consider them mine. From the first day of pregnancy, even from the moment I made up my mind that I'd carry my daughter's children, I realized they were someone else's. I felt them kicking inside me and I just laughed. I enjoyed and loved the feeling of them but I didn't experience any strong maternal instincts or urges.

When I first heard the babies cry in the operating

theatre it was just beautiful. They sounded so cute. I felt like any other happy granny whose daughter had just had a child. I don't even feel that these lovely grandchildren of mine have ever been inside me. Although they will always be special to me I was only the incubator in which they grew.

And as she lay recovering in her hospital bed, Pat went on:

I did all this because of my daughter, because she, not I, was desperate for more children. She was unhappy and I have tried to make her happy.

It has been a total commitment for almost a year of my life and I feel great about having done it. Karen and Alcino have now got themselves a nice family. I never considered what I was doing was anything really different. I just did what I hope any mother would do for a daughter who was deprived of having children.

The same morning of the birth, when David was just three hours old, Karen put the first-born of the triplets to her breast. It was a moving moment and one that the 25-year-old had looked forward to for many, many months. 'I put him to my right breast and he sucked and sucked straight away. I could hear him swallowing for about five minutes and I know he got quite a bit of milk. Then he gave a nice big burp.' It was an important breakthrough for Karen and made all her hard work preparing to produce milk worthwhile. Since arriving in Johannesburg to be with her mother during the pregnancy, she had been using a breast pump three times a day.

That same morning Karen bathed David, in the intensive care unit where Jose and Paula were still in incubators to keep them warm. It would be some two weeks before the tiniest of the trio would come off an intravenous feed, because she was so small. Those first days were filled with joy as Karen got to know her babies, their little whims and their individual characters. David was impatient, she was to declare, Jose a good boy who fed well. Paula, who had still not been held for any length of time by her mother, was still an unknown quantity, but the exact image of Karen.

Within 36 hours of the birth Pat was well enough to visit her grandchildren. And on the afternoon of 2 October she was again put in a wheelchair and taken down the corridor, dressed in a smart maroon dressing-gown, to see them for the very first time. Again this remarkable grandmother was to surprise all those who had doubted she would be able to relinquish the babies, all those who had predicted that she would be in mental anguish at the sight of the children she must never call her very own. As one by one the babies were placed in her arms, she smiled proudly but was quick to turn to Karen and ask for the little details that only a mother knows. 'Does he feed well now?' she questioned her daughter of the baby David. 'Isn't she small?' she said of Paula. It must have been a relief to Karen to see her mother acting like any grandmother the world over.

There was no hint of jealousy, no indication that Pat would ever regret her amazing act of generosity. Indeed Pat's main thoughts now related to when she could leave the clinic and begin her life again. After a month in one room she was making plans to holiday on the Durban coast with Raymond and was becoming irritated with the hospital routine, the strictures of the nurses about her need to rest after the operation, and above all the limits of the hospital food.

But Pat had another obstacle to cross although she did not know it then. Alarmingly, four days after the birth, her temperature soared inexplicably. This immediately curtailed her short visits down the corridor to see the three triplets and her path to recovery. At first no one knew what was wrong with Pat, who because of the sudden illness became depressed and tearful in a way that was quite out of character. Some nurses on ward three were quick to blame the post-natal blues for her low spirits, but Pat indignantly denied this was the cause of her anguish.

She lay in a darkened room in the Park Lane Clinic for 24

hours but her temperature did not come down. And it was only after Dr Michelow had been alerted about her high temperature that the true cause of her ailment was discovered. This was not the baby blues but the flaring up of a minor internal infection.

When Pat had undergone the Caesarian operation a tiny fragment of the afterbirth had been left behind to fester inside her body. Dr Michelow immediately made arrangements for his important patient to be readmitted to the operating theatre next morning for an exploratory operation. As a precaution the doctors decided that the operation would not take place in the surgical wing of the Park Lane Clinic, which would entail Pat being wheeled in her bed right through the hospital building, past the watching and wondering nurses, doctors and patients. Instead she would go into the same labour ward operating theatre where she had so successfully given birth to the triplets.

Dr Michelow performed a D and C (dilation and curettage) on Pat Anthony to clean out her womb, a simple and straightforward operation which took less than half an hour on 7 October. By 11 o'clock that morning Pat was sleeping back in her room, her temperature immediately down and her recovery started again. It was a tremendous relief to everyone, especially her loving family. For while the three babies were now really beginning to thrive, it would have been a horrible tragedy if anything had been allowed to jeopardize the health of their grandmother.

Despite the efforts to keep the operation on Pat a secret as she herself wished, rumours abounded in the hospital. In the first crucial days after the birth Pat had tried to walk, taking slow steps around the hospital room with the helping arm of Raymond around her. At first she had had trouble standing up straight, but following the operation she had quickly become more sprightly, more like the Pat of old who would run rather than walk down the main street of Tzaneen in her hurry to get from one point to another in double-quick time.

Within 24 hours of the trip to the labour ward theatre a

bystander would have noticed nothing amiss about Pat Anthony. Remarkably, she recovered so fast that very soon she was making her own way down the hospital corridor unaided and needed no help from the nurses to slip to the bathroom during the night. Now her main ambition was to get home as swiftly as possible, to move out from the confines of the hospital.

By eight days after the birth Pat was telling the astounded doctors that she must leave the hospital. She brooked no opposition to her plan and asked Raymond to be ready to pick her up at the clinic on Sunday morning. She wanted to join him at his Johannesburg hotel and then go out to Sunday lunch at Mandy and Cliffie Jacob's home. Every minute she seemed to grow stronger and with persistence she finally persuaded the medical team and her own family that it was time to say goodbye to the hospital.

On that Sunday morning Pat planned to pay a last visit to her three very special grandchildren. She dressed carefully in a midnight-blue silk dress and neat, low-heeled beige shoes. No one could have guessed this woman had just given birth to triplets. Her weight was only five pounds above what she had tipped the scales at ten months before. To be sure, her waistline for the time being was not what it had been, but Pat, who had always watched her figure, was confident that with exercise this would soon return to normal.

She walked down the ward three corridor out to the intensive care unit where Karen was feeding the babies. And there she behaved like any caring grandmother. The eldest triplet, David, was protesting with a small baby's howls about having the bottle put to his mouth by Karen. He turned his head away and yowled so much that Pat could not stop herself offering some advice. 'That baby has had too much milk already,' she warned her worried daughter with a smile. 'I am telling you, Karen, that he doesn't want any more to eat at the moment.' The words, although not designed to interfere, would have irritated the most devoted of daughters trying to cope with a newborn baby. Karen responded by raising her eyes to the ceiling and retorting, 'OK, Ma, it is me here who is doing the feeding, not you'.

The incident was not an important one. It was the sort of scene that happens in every family. But it served to show how very normal the relationship between Pat and her grandchildren was from the very beginning. Here she was behaving like a grandmother without any soul-searching about her role in the triplets' life.

Yet sadly the South African press was again to distort the truth about what Pat Anthony felt about her grandchildren and her recovery after the historic birth. That very morning, as Pat admired the babies and watched Karen feeding them, the *Sunday Star* of Johannesburg had published a front-page article which made chilling reading.

'Granny is a Broken Woman,' yelled the headline. 'She looks as though she has had 10 children, never mind triplets.' The article went on to insist that Pat Anthony, the Tzaneen surrogate granny, was 'over the hill'.

It read: 'Doubts were expressed in the medical world this week about the wisdom of allowing a 48-year-old woman to carry triplets. Some doctors are reported as saying the physical and emotional strain would be severe.' And the article added: 'Fears about the health of her mother and that of her fragile daughter, Paula, the tiniest of the triplets, are ageing 25-year-old Karen.'

The words were cruel enough and the fact that they were totally without foundation made them no less cutting to the family. Only Pat laughed at the article, because as she said, 'How can I take these lies seriously?'

Ironically, after leaving the hospital that Sunday morning Pat walked down the long corridor of the Johannesburg hotel where she and Raymond were to stay for a week. Outside each bedroom door was a copy of the Johannesburg *Sunday Star*, delivered free to hotel guests as a courtesy. Staring up at Pat was the headline 'Granny is a Broken Woman'. She marched past each door and each newspaper without flinching. It was indicative of her whole attitude to the event that had stunned the world. For Pat the family came first and as long as Karen had three healthy babies and she could go home to Tzaneen with Raymond, then nothing else mattered at all.

Yet Pat wondered why the South African press were so hostile to her and the family's decision to give their story to a London newspaper. After all, she reasoned, the South African premier newspaper – the Johannesburg *Sunday Times* – had back in March 1987 been offered the story exclusively in a telephone call to their offices by Alcino. But this newspaper had turned it down flat.

In Tzaneen, where Pat would return in another fortnight, there was already a welcome waiting. For the triplets by chance had been born on the birthday of the town's mayor, Mr Johan van Vuuren. And if some member of the South African press chose to snipe at the event, the citizens of Tzaneen cared not a jot. They would only celebrate more thoroughly the birth that had put the Transvaal fruit-growing area on the map. Mr Vuuren, contacted by the South African glossy magazine, *Personality*, on the day of the birth, had said:

I personally think what Pat Anthony has done is tremendous. It takes guts as well as love and if you know Pat you will understand why she did it. She and her whole family are kind, soft-hearted people. Not only are the grandparents paying all their own expenses but they don't want to receive one cent themselves. Any money the family receive for interviews will be put into a trust fund for the three children.

The family is very popular in Tzaneen because they are all such likeable people. They own an up-market interior decorating shop which does very well. The whole town is proud of Pat and the family.

Just as the telegrams and flowers had flooded into the hospital after the birth, now letters were being sent to Tzaneen from all over the globe from ordinary people who had read Pat's amazing story. One of the hundreds to arrive in the little town post office said: 'Dear Mr Postman. Please find the surrogate granny from Tzaneen, South Africa, and make sure she gets this letter.' It came all the way from Australia and was delivered to Pat's front door soon after she returned to the town.

Now the dust had settled Pat and Karen were only worried about one thing. In South Africa's corridors of power there had been constant rumblings for two months about exactly who the triplets would belong to once they were born. The Government's Justice Minister Kobie Coetsee indicated that planned changes in the country's laws meant that because she had borne them, the triplets would belong to Pat Anthony. Although Karen was the children's biological mother, in law she would be seen as their sister because the Act, passed two weeks after the birth, now declared that in cases of surrogacy all ties between the biological mother and the unborn child should be severed.

It was a complicated issue and although Mr Coetsee had spoken out, the law itself had never been actually tested. So the family, with the help of the Park Lane Clinic and Vita Lab doctors, decided to take a risk. If the new legislation really meant that Pat was the children's mother, and not their grandmother, because she had given birth to them, then Karen would be forced to adopt her own three babies. And this was exactly what the family did not want.

So, without much ado, Dr Michelow and Matron Groat devised a special form of words to be put on the birth registration form which the hospital had to fill in within seven days of any birth. The form read that David, Jose and Paula had been born 'of Karen Ferreira-Jorge' but 'by Pat Anthony'.

With any luck this might be accepted by the South African Department of the Interior which would make the final decision about exactly who was the mother of the triplets. There was no precedent to rely on for there had never been a surrogate birth in South Africa before. When the form arrived at the Department of the Interior the officials would never have seen anything like it. The question was would these South African bureaucrats, many of them members of the disapproving Dutch Reformed Church, accept the unconventional wording on the form and issue a birth certificate naming Karen as mother?

'Although Mrs Anthony has made it clear that she is willing to give up the triplets, which are apparently legally her children, for adoption by their sister, the permutations have all the makings of a music-hall comic's joke,' commented one civil law expert when approached by the magazine *Personality* about the tangle. But as a psychologist told the same magazine, 'Fortunately, Pat Anthony seemed never to have regarded the children as her own. However emotional ties do develop between a woman and a child which grows in her womb and any surrogate mother could be strongly tempted to retain the offspring she bears, particularly when the law seems to indicate they are hers.'

It would be another two months before the family were told if the babies were to be Karen's own or belong to Pat: two months of anxiety for this mother and daughter.

Chapter 9

The next days were long ones for Karen Ferreira-Jorge as she lived at the Park Lane Clinic with the three new babies. The boys, David and Jose, had put on weight and were ready to go home but little Paula was still in the intensive care unit, progressing well but not yet sturdy enough to leave the hospital.

While Karen stayed on in her room, the boys would be brought to her each morning and she would spend the day with them. It was her first chance to devote time to David and Jose like any other mother. Meanwhile she would feed Paula every four hours, supplementing her breast milk with the bottle, knowing the doctors would not let her daughter go back to Tzaneen and the waiting yellow nursery until she was two kilos (4.40 lbs) in weight.

Alcino Senior had already returned to his job as a refrigeration engineer in Tzaneen, taking with him Alcino Junior who had coped so well with the arrival of his two new brothers and sister. Before the birth little Alcino had boasted that his brothers and sister were growing in his grandmother's tummy because his own mummy had no room in her own. Now he was calling David, Jose and Paula 'his babies', and showed – much to Karen's relief – no signs of jealousy about the triplets.

Already press interest in the Tzaneen family was abating, especially as Pat had left the hospital. But each day the Park Lane Clinic switchboard and the Matron, Beverley Frieslich, would fend off calls from the local newspapers about exactly when Karen would be going home with the babies.

'It was a lonely time,' says Karen now, 'especially with none of my family with me. But it was important too because I had the chance to get the boys into some sort of routine. They got to know me as I got to know them. Yet I was itching to get everyone home at last.'

In the intensive care unit Paula began to put on weight well but Karen found the baby crotchety at feeding time.

> She was difficult to deal with because she was so small and kept going to sleep. Although I didn't produce much milk I found she was comforted if I put her to my breast. We began to build up a bond together but much more slowly than the boys, mainly because for the first few weeks Paula had been tended by the specially trained nurses rather than me.

But by Saturday 31 October, a month after the birth, Paula's weight had climbed to 1.9 kilos and Dr Michelow, with the paediatrician Maxwell Hopp, decided that she was strong enough to make the 300-mile journey to Tzaneen with Karen, home to the Ferreira-Jorge house for the first time.

That morning, although little had been said in the hospital about the homegoing, the South African press congregated outside the clinic hoping for a picture of Karen with three white bundles, but this was not to be. While Alcino Senior occupied the journalists at the front of the building a plan was mounted by Matron Frieslich to get the rest of the family away unhindered. Carrying the babies in their arms, Karen and the matron travelled by lift down through the inside of the building and took a back route to the car park past the hospital mortuary. Then in the matron's car they drove to a rendezvous in the Parktown suburb where

Alcino Senior waited in a combie van borrowed for the occasion from a friend.

'First we went to Mandy Jacob's home to feed the babies ready for the five-hour journey. We were worried at the time about how they would cope with the travelling but they slept most of the way,' says Karen. 'It was different when we finally got home though.'

In the townhouse nursery, with its jolly cartoons of Mickey Mouse and Donald Duck on the walls, the babies woke Karen and Alcino persistently throughout the first two nights. 'We didn't sleep at all,' remembers Alcino Senior now. Then he jokes, 'I began to wish they had never been born at all'.

During the days immediately after the family's arrival back in Tzaneen they were beseiged by well-meaning locals, sympathetic mothers, friends, relatives and even total strangers. All wanted to have a look at the babies and some visitors even arrived uninvited at 7.30 in the morning. 'Everyone was very inquisitive but I didn't mind at all apart from those who literally just knocked on the door and walked in before breakfast as though we were a public peep show,' Karen said.

Very soon it became obvious that if Karen was to enjoy her babies and their first few months of life a night nurse was needed. 'From the moment she came I was able to sleep and not be so exhausted during the daytime. We began to operate like a proper family although I hardly sat down at all during the day unless I had a baby in one arm and a bottle in the other.'

At first Karen rarely took the babies out into the town, but gradually she became accustomed to popping one in the car with her when she went shopping. 'I took it in turns, one baby one day and another the next. It was nice for them to be away from the other two for a change. It also gave me a chance to be alone with one of the triplets.'

Pat was now back from her holiday in Port Shepstone with Raymond. Immediately she went to work again, helping in the shop and doing the accounts for the gift business which had been put to one side in the run-up to the birth and its immediate aftermath. 'I didn't have time to convalesce or just sit at home,' she recalls today. 'You won't believe it, but I was so busy that I sometimes didn't see the triplets for a week in the early days.'

But when Pat did visit Karen's house, with its white nappies flapping on the railings around the communal swimming pool, she was nervous about handling the babies who had grown inside her. From the distance of a comfortable armchair she commented, 'I can't believe I carried these three babies. I feel worried now if one cries or even hiccups. I am glad it is Karen, not me, who is having to cope.'

It would amaze most outsiders just how contentedly the family settled back into their normal lives, after a year in the constant blaze of publicity. Now only one thing worried them. All through October and November they had heard nothing from the Department of the Interior about who would be deemed to be the mother of the triplets. With the birth not yet properly registered, no plans could be made about having the children christened as Roman Catholics, which had been the earnest wish of both Karen and Pat from the very beginning.

While newspapers and television stations in South Africa no longer carried long daily items about the family and the famous surrogate granny, it seemed unlikely to Karen and Alcino Senior that the Dutch Reformed Church, to which so many of the Department of the Interior's ministers and civil servants belonged, could change its view of the birth. This Church's leading intellectuals had publicly deemed the event 'unsavoury' and its policy dictated that surrogate motherhood was wrong.

Night after night Karen and Alcino Senior would discuss the dilemma, concerned above all that they should not have to adopt the children who were biologically theirs and already looked like their mother and father. It was a testing time and Pat too was worried about her position if the babies were legally declared her offspring. 'These are

Karen and Alcino Senior's children and I was only the vessel to carry them,' she would repeat to anyone who quizzed her on that delicate matter.

But early in December, a few weeks before Christmas, the registration forms were returned from the Pretoria Government offices naming Karen as the triplets' mother. No comment was made by officialdom, no explanation was offered for the decision. Now there would be no need for tortuous legal battles or lengthy adoption procedures and it was a day for celebration.

Yet, although the family did not realize it then, the chances of the babies being recognized as Karen's had been very, very slim. And if many experienced lawyers in South Africa had been asked for their views on the registration of the births, they would have said it should never have happened.

For on 14 October 1987, a fortnight after the triplets came into the world, South Africa enacted a new Children's Status Act which declared that any baby born to a married woman who has had artificial insemination with the consent of her husband is deemed to be the legitimate offspring of that married couple.

If that law was retrospective, as some of South Africa's most prominent advocates say it was, then Pat Anthony should have been named the mother of the children as a married woman who had undergone artificial insemination of ova and semen with the consent of her husband.

But luckily for Karen and Alcino the registration was allowed to go ahead although there are those who warn today that this was illegal. One expert on surrogacy, Professor Louise Tager, Professor of Law at the University of Witwatersrand has commented:

> When the Children's Status Act was drafted, I don't believe it was realized that it would affect surrogate arrangements, such as Mrs Pat Anthony's.
>
> But it so happened that it was worded in such a way that it did cover this type of surrogacy, although it was

designed to address the problem of illegitimate children born by artificial insemination.

'Right from the beginning we decided to play the whole business of registering the births in a very low-key way,' says Alcino today. 'We did not provoke the authorities by making statements about what we thought should happen. We just sent in the registration forms in the normal way but saying the babies were born of Karen Ferreira-Jorge by Pat Anthony.'

Immediately Karen started planning the christening at the Tzaneen Roman Catholic Church and when David, Jose and Paula were three months old, on Karen's 26th birthday on 22 January 1988, they were quietly baptized in the church where their parents had married and the family had worshipped over the years.

It was a simple enough ceremony, attended by only their closest friends and relatives. Yet the event was a tribute to the family's determination and the understanding of their local priest, who by conducting the christening at all denied the Pope's strict rulings outlawing *in-vitro* fertilization and surrogacy.

From the very beginning the family had consulted their parish priest, Father Sean Laffan, about their hopes of Pat bearing the children for her barren daughter. And although leading Roman Catholic churchmen in South Africa had declared openly once the pregnancy became public that any children born as a result of it should not be christened, Father Laffan had promised that the babies would be treated the same as any others in his small community.

It was brave of Father Laffan who from April 1987 onwards had been confronted with publicity about the conflict between surrogacy and the dictates of the Roman Catholic Church. A typical news item at the time quoted the respected lecturer in moral theology at St John Vianney Seminary, Pretoria, a Father Hyacinth Ennie, as declaring:

The Vatican has said conception other than through natural sexual acts between married couples is morally illicit. It is contrary to the unity of marriage and to the dignity of the procreation of the human person. The question of marriage itself is involved as surrogacy involves the introduction of a third party.

Father Hyacinth was not alone in publicly condemning what this Roman Catholic family planned to do. But Father Laffan only asked Karen that the christening should not become a target for newspaper publicity and his condition was adhered to by the grateful family, who kept all details of the christening secret from all but the six godparents.

The two baby boys were dressed in white romper suits, bought by Pat in the Tzaneen children's boutique. Paula was adorned in a matching full-length gown, a gift from her godmother, Mandy Jacob. 'It was a very important day for us all,' recalls Karen today. 'We are practising Roman Catholics and it was deeply satisfying to know that our babies had been admitted into the Church despite what the Pope had said about surrogate births. Pat, in particular, has always believed that their conception and safe arrival was a gift from God. It made her very happy.'

On that happy afternoon, Pat, Raymond and Alcino Junior watched as the water was poured on each of the triplets' heads, Father Laffan only fluffing his lines once or twice by saying child, instead of children, as though he was christening one baby and not three. Paula made the family laugh by protesting most loudly when the water touched her while Jose slept through the whole afternoon, unaware of his admission to the Roman Catholic Church.

The family believed so strongly that the triplets should be christened into the Church, that Alcino Senior had even started plans to take his children to his parents' home in Portugal for the baptism to take place. There, in Europe and many miles away, there would be less controversy and no one would even know the origins of the children. But thankfully, because of Father Laffan, this would not now be necessary.

Back in their Tzaneen home, Karen and Alcino threw a little tea party with three christening cakes on display, one for each of the babies. The six godparents were there and just as any other day of the week neighbours and friends called in, popping out again past the nappies hanging on the fence outside. By now Karen was washing 30 nappies a day with the help of her loyal black maid, Sabena. It was hard work at the beginning but there have been many moments of joy for this young mother during the first year of her babies' lives.

Paula, who nearly died before even being born, was at five months old the first triplet to roll herself over without a helping hand. It was a triumphant moment for a child who was still underweight for her age because of the premature birth. She would, the family predicted, become the first of the trio to crawl as well.

Paula looks like Karen and has grown close to her mother.

> One day, well after I had stopped breast-feeding the babies, Paula was niggling and refusing to take to the bottle. I put her to my breast, although she was beginning to teethe by this stage. Immediately she became contented and fell asleep. I felt that we now really knew each other well.

Alcino Junior has been going to nursery school in the mornings on the outskirts of Tzaneen, and very soon he will begin primary school. Alcino Senior comes home in the evenings to take a share of the bottle-feeding but as Karen says somewhat ruefully, 'As yet I have never managed to persuade him to change a nappy. Perhaps he will when they grow older.'

In March the family moved from their neat but tiny townhouse to a four-bedroomed home with a big garden where Alcino and the triplets will be able to play and run in safety. Because of the night nurse there has been no need to call on Pat to babysit yet but when Karen and Alcino Senior were househunting they asked Raymond to watch over the babies for an hour one afternoon.

'It is a bit of a family joke,' laughs Karen today. 'The babies were all asleep when we left them with my father at his house. But we hadn't been away one minute when one by one they each woke up and cried. They kept that up for the hour. He hasn't offered to have them again.'

Anecdotes like this serve to illustrate how well this remarkable family from a small, remote town in the depths of the South African countryside have adjusted back to normal once outside the intense public gaze. Together they have emeged unscathed from their year of dealings with the world's press, the South African government, the Dutch Reformed Church, the Roman Catholic Church and doctors at the forefront of the reproduction revolution.

Pat herself seems to have survived it all particularly well. Only her husband Raymond is more cynical about the future and what it holds for the family. He faced the brunt of the press scramble for information when Pat was first pregnant and hidden away in Johannesburg. He alone had to cope with the battalions of reporters trying to track down their quarry. He is the only man in the world to know what it is like to see your wife pregnant with your daughter and son-in-law's baby.

> I have had to force myself to forget the hostility towards the surrogate birth and Pat from some quarters, including the South African press, the Dutch Reformed Church and even the government. I am trying to put all that behind me and remember that we have achieved exactly what we set out to do so long ago: give Karen the children she couldn't have herself.

But now, every day and all day, Raymond is reminded of 1987 and the year he became the grandfather of three surrogate triplets who had been carried by his wife.

> People come into the shop and ask for half a yard of ribbon, and then say how are the triplets? It is the same with every customer, every person I bump into out in the street, every caller at my home. Therefore I know life will never really be the same again.

Already he realizes that whatever happens to the family, from a wedding to job promotion, will always front-page news in South Africa. 'I nearly bumped into another car the other day,' remembers Raymond. 'I came very close to it indeed then I thought afterwards it would have caused mayhem. It would not have been deemed a simple crash because I am the grandfather of the triplets. My picture and their pictures would have been all over the television.'

Raymond, like the rest of the family, is aware too that if any of the triplets get involved in any event which is even very slightly out of the ordinary, be it a playground scuffle or a learning problem, this too may provoke a newspaper or television story.

> I hope this doesn't make us over-protective of them. The trouble is that inevitably their babyhood has already been shared by so many people out there, and their childhood, teenage and adult lives are likely to be the same. For now ordinary people, especially those here in Tzaneen, see these children as 'their triplets'. Now I am almost afraid if one of them catches a cold.

But as for David, Jose and Paula, they will be brought up as their parents were brought up. Their devoted mother and father will tell them that family life is important, that the sanctity of marriage is absolute and about caring for others. And if that in 1988 sounds old-fashioned, it is still very much current thinking in the small Lebanese community in Tzaneen, South Africa. Very soon, as soon as they can understand such things, they will be told that their grandmother was the person who carried them for nine months in her womb. They will be told about the very special gift of love that their grandmother gave to her daughter, their mother Karen. These three children will learn how much they were yearned for and how they were welcomed by their family on the morning of an October day in 1987.

They are now unique, but perhaps when they grow up they will not be the only children in the world to have been borne by their own grandmother. By then, with medical science advancing so fast, the concept of a mother carrying her daughter's baby may not be unusual.

As Alcino Senior so sensibly says:

> Science plays a huge part in everyone's lives these days. Technical developments have brought huge achievements in all areas. This is simply an extension of that and like every new development it takes time for people to stop being frightened, as they were for instance when they first travelled on steam trains.

Chapter 10

The law surrounding surrogacy is complex. Yet in all the countries at the forefront of test-tube baby-making and surrogacy, legislation is slowly being enacted to cover this expanding area of medical science. But as the Melbourne daily newspaper, *The Age*, put it in an editorial back in August 1981:

> Like the hare and the tortoise, science and the law run a permanently unequal race. While science moves in dazzling leaps and pirouettes, weaving wonder and miracles, the law plods sedately behind and collects the dust. It is sometimes a very long plod.

In Britain it was not until the autumn of 1987 that the government's White Paper on embryo research and surrogacy was finally published. It said, as the Warnock Committee had recommended, that a childless couple who enter into an arrangement with a surrogate should have no legal rights over the baby that is born. Furthermore any surrogacy contract should be unenforceable in the courts of law. The recommendations, if accepted by parliament, will give surrogate mothers the absolute right to keep any child or children they bear; a stipulation which will probably deter most barren couples from using surrogacy as a way of starting a family. The same White Paper made it clear that any woman who bears a child after artificial insemination by donor or embryo donation will also be its legal mother.

Although the government's White Paper did not outlaw surrogacy arrangements, other than those by commercial agencies, its decision to give the surrogate mother all legal rights to the child will make it virtually impossible for the commissioning parents to adopt the child if the carrying mother does not wish this to happen.

The White Paper was unequivocal too about non-commercial agencies promoting surrogate arrangements. It insisted that they should not be given licences and, again, any contract they entered into on behalf of others would have no legal standing in the courts. However it did not propose to alter the Surrogacy Arrangements Act 1985 rushed through following the birth of Baby Cotton. This said that the surrogate mother and the commissioning parents should be free from prosecution even when the arrangement is made through a commercial agency.

The White Paper stated:

> We do not at present propose to extend the criminal law any further in this field of surrogacy but intend that a statutory licensing authority should be asked to examine the whole practice of surrogacy so that parliament can review the situation from time to time on the basis of informed advice.

At the same time the government took the opportunity to propose tougher controls over test-tube fertilization and clinics involved with the highly controversial embryo research. A complete ban on genetic manipulation of human embryos was put forward.

Under the White Paper's suggestions, it would become a criminal offence to use spare embryos obtained during the test-tube baby treatments for research into cloning or genetic alteration. Scientists involved in embryo research would now have to demonstrate that this research would lead to improvements in the treatment of congenital disease, the detection of gene or chromosome abnormalities, or the advancement of contraception.

Any experiments, said the government, must be monitored by a statutory licensing authority.

> One of the greatest causes of public concern has been the perceived possibility that newly developed techniques will allow the artificial creation of human beings with certain predetermined characteristics.
>
> The technical prospects for achieving this are in fact extremely remote. Nevertheless it is a procedure which society would clearly regard as ethically unacceptable and the Bill will prohibit it.

Controversially, the White Paper included two alternative draft clauses – one making it a criminal offence to carry out any embryo research and the other permitting licensed research projects – indicating the government's view that the issue is a matter of individual conscience.

Opponents of research argue that from the point of conception, embryos have the same status as a child or an adult and it is improper to conduct research, whatever its benefits for others, that would lead to the destruction of that embryo. Those who favour the continuation of embryo research argue that it offers very important benefits, for example, in detecting genetic disorders.

Immediately the White Paper was published doctors began to put forward their views on its contents. Professor Robert Winston, head of the infertility clinic at London's Hammersmith Hospital, said that the White Paper rightly reflected the deep concern that some people had over this research. 'However,' he told *The Times* of London on 27 November 1987, 'I am concerned that the public should be aware that embryologists and research workers are on the brink of an enormous breakthrough in the prevention of hereditary and genetic diseases.'

The anti-abortion pressure group, Life, applauded the fact that the government had left to a free vote the alternative clauses, one prohibiting any research and the other allowing a limited degree of research on embryos. The Life lobby declared at this time that it believed a majority of MPs in the House of Commons would vote against any research in this controversial and sensitive field.

In America new legislation is being drawn up to cover surrogacy. In February 1988 a panel of specialists based in Philadelphia concluded that payments to surrogate mothers for bearing a child should be prohibited, even when this involved a loss of parental rights. The panel of lawyers, physicians and ethicists also ruled that surrogate contracts made before conception should be unenforceable in the courts and fees to brokers, some of whom in the US have grown rich from this trade, must be prohibited.

A member of the panel was Barbara Shack, a member of the New York civil liberties union board who is co-ordinator for the New York Coalition for Choice. As she says, 'If payment of money is contingent upon giving up the baby, that's baby-selling.'

A few days before that panel met the New Jersey Supreme Court reached the same conclusion on payment to surrogate mothers, a decision that invalidated the contract between Mary Beth Whitehead, the surrogate in the Baby M case, and William and Elizabeth Stern. Mary Beth was artificially impregnated with the sperm of William Stern (see page 67) and under the contract would have been required to turn over her daughter to this man and his wife in return for 10,000 dollars. As it is, Mary Beth now has visiting rights and successfully appealed for more time with the child she gave birth to, although the Sterns have custody of the baby now known as Melissa.

All of America looked to this vital ruling because surrogacy laws there evolve state by state. The New Jersey judges held that surrogacy transactions, like those in the Baby M case, were simply illegal baby-selling under their own state legislation and also 'perhaps criminal and potentially degrading to the women involved'.

Elsewhere in America the clampdown on surrogacy is

now well underway. In Lincoln, Nebraska on 5 February 1988 a new bill was approved to declare surrogate motherhood contracts void. It was passed by a significant majority of 41 votes to 1. The lone dissenter was State Senator Shirley March, who said she was concerned that childless couples would no longer have the option of surrogacy open to them. Early in 1988 the Connecticut General Assembly's judiciary committee was working on a proposal to ban all surrogate agreements. The proposer of this move was Richard Tulisano, a Democrat who tried to introduce a similar bill three years before.

But not every area of the United States is taking the same very hard line on surrogacy. Noel P. Keane is a lawyer who operates an infertility clinic in Dearborn, Michigan and is still receiving dozens of calls daily from the anguished infertile who need help. Mr Keane originated the first surrogate motherhood contracts in 1976 and was instrumental in bringing together Mary Beth Whitehead and the Sterns.

On the walls of his New York Office there are dozens of pictures of babies born through surrogacy. He has introduced 200 childless couples to women prepared to act as surrogates for a 10,000 dollar fee plus medical expenses.

Mr Keane claims that of the 500 or 600 babies born to surrogate mothers in the United States over the last decade there have been only five cases where the baby has not been handed over to the commissioning parents. This, he points out, is a tiny, tiny proportion of those who have used surrogacy to have the babies they crave.

In Michigan a 16-member panel of doctors, lawyers and, perhaps most importantly, the clergy has met to discuss the 'reproductive technologies' and has not recommended the complete outlawing of surrogacy. Only the production of babies for money-making or the payment of a fee beyond reasonable expenses should be banned, said this panel.

But in California, the legislature in 1986 killed off a forward-thinking new bill spelling out in detail how surrogacy contracts should be drawn up and how they could be made to work within necessary safeguards. Then Assemblyman Elija Harris, a Democrat, complained: 'The issues are so confusing that the legislators have chosen not to address themselves to this problem at this time.'

In Australia, where much of the early work on test-tube conception took place, fee-paying surrogacy is slowly being outlawed too. As in America, it is on a state by state basis. Ahead of the game is Victoria which has had a specific ban on commercial surrogacy for four years. In 1988 two other states, Queensland and South Australia, were planning to bring in legislation to ban surrogacies for monetary return. In other states, namely New South Wales, Western Australia, the Northern Territory and Tasmania, there is no legislation covering contracts for surrogate motherhood. But the law states that money cannot be exchanged for babies under any circumstances, a measure that effectively stops commercial surrogacy deals of any kind.

These moves to control surrogate motherhood are underway despite a public opinion poll conducted in May 1987 which showed that more than half of all Australians, male and female, support surrogacy as a method of helping the infertile have the children they want so badly.

The new poll, believed to be the first in the world on surrogate motherhood, consisted of a national survey of 2,500 people and was organized by the New South Wales Law Reform Commission. At the time the Commission was collecting evidence before deciding on changes to laws covering artificial conception. The survey found that 51 per cent of people were in favour of, or did not oppose, surrogate motherhood. Another 33 per cent of those questioned disapproved of surrogacy and 13 per cent had no opinion whatsoever on this most contentious of issues.

Most of the Australians questioned believed the surrogate mother should be paid for carrying the child of another couple; 40 per cent favoured paying the surrogate mother her medical expenses plus an agreed fee for her time and trouble, while 34 per cent thought only her medical costs should be met.

The poll considered the question of who should be able to claim the baby if there was a dispute between the infertile commissioning couple and the surrogate mother. One person in three thought the baby in this case should be handed to the couple, while 25 per cent believed that the surrogate mother should keep the child. A further 25 per cent said that a court of law must decide on this issue.

After the poll was conducted, the Law Reform Commission deputy chairman, Mr Russell Scott, said that between 10 per cent and 15 per cent of Australian couples were infertile, a fact that in theory makes artificial conception an important issue for one million Australians.

'There has been so much knee-jerk government reaction to this question,' commented Mr Scott. 'In 1984 Victoria passed this law, making surrogate motherhood an offence when any money is involved. No other country in the world took such harsh action so early.'

The Victorian Government's decision followed an investigation by Professor Louis Waller into the whole of the test-tube baby programme in this particular state. The Waller report strongly opposed the practice of surrogate motherhood and as a result Victoria decided to ban payments for surrogate motherhood arrangements and to make surrogacy contracts unenforceable in the courts. Britain now looks poised to follow suit.

The Victorian Government also decided to make it an offence to place or publish an advertisement for a surrogate mother, or for a potential surrogate mother to offer her services to an infertile couple.

Queensland's fresh legislation will also make it illegal to advertise to recruit women for surrogate pregnancies or to provide facilities for people who wish to make use of the services of such women. Dr John Hennessey, a Queensland physician and fertility expert, is one who approves these moves. 'Several childless couples have approached me and my colleagues in the hope of obtaining a baby through a surrogate mother. But I have said that for a woman to give up her baby puts her under terrible emotional strain and I have always been against it.'

South Australia proposes to make surrogate motherhood contracts unenforceable and the state's health ministry has said that any fee paid to a person organizing a surrogacy contract will be recoverable by the couple who paid the fee.

Dr John Porter, of Melbourne's Infertility Medical Centre, has said that while there must be legal protection for some kinds of surrogacy, a case can be made for the continuation of non-commercial arrangements where no money passes hands.

But he pointed out that doctors in Melbourne, where test-tube baby-making was pioneered, no longer felt confident about taking an egg from an infertile woman, fertilizing it and placing it in a surrogate mother's uterus in the present legal and ethical climate.

Mrs Maria Gold, secretary of the Australia's *in-vitro* fertilization patient support group, has spoken out about the 'very big difference' between commercial and non-commercial surrogacy. 'Children must not be bought, but when the mother does not get paid we don't see it as an ethical problem.' She is not alone in believing that surrogacy should be allowed to survive, but the state governments of Australia are taking a much more conservative attitude to the new ways of baby-making which have sprung up courtesy of science.

Ironically South Africa, where Pat Anthony gave birth to her daughter's children on 1 October 1987, has lagged behind in legislating for all kinds of surrogate baby-bearing. This country's lateness in pronouncing on the legality of surrogacy may well be because until the birth of the Ferreira-Jorge triplets there had never been a surrogacy in South Africa for the legislators to consider or pronounce about.

But when Pat Anthony was three months into her pregnancy, the South African press revealed the government's plans to introduce a new law called the Children's Status Act. The Act aimed to clear up confusion about the legal status of children conceived by artificial insemination, yet would have the effect of making any surrogate mother the legal parent of the child born to her.

The relevant clause in the Act stipulated that a baby conceived by artificial insemination was the legal offspring of the woman who gave birth to it and her husband if they were married. A memo on the objects of the Bill explained: 'All legal ties between the child and outsiders are also severed.'

The Bill was enacted on 14 October 1987 – the same day as the Ferreira-Jorge triplets were due to be born and a fortnight after they actually came into the world. In the event after two anxious months for the family (see page 106) the birth of the triplets was registered with Alcino and Karen Ferreira-Jorge confirmed as their parents.

But there are some leading South African lawyers who now say that the Children's Status Act was designed to be retrospective. If that is the case then Pat Anthony should have been named as the mother of the triplets and the births could never have been registered in the way they were. Instead Alcino and Karen should have adopted the three babies.

Louise Tager, Professor of Law at Witwatersrand University, Cape Town has made a detailed study of the legal implications of surrogacy and artificial insemination in South Africa and across the world. An advocate of the Supreme Court of South Africa, she explains:

> Until 1987, before the Children's Status Act was passed, any child born as a result of artificial insemination by donor was illegitimate, even if the husband consented to his wife being inseminated in this way. The husband had to adopt the child later to make it legitimate and rightly his own.
>
> The Children's Status Act changed the legal effect of artificial insemination. It ruled that whenever a married woman has had artificial insemination – and that includes *in-vitro* fertilization – with the consent of her

husband (as Mrs Pat Anthony did), any children born as a result are deemed to be the legitimate children of that married couple.

The argument about whether the Ferreira-Jorge triplets should have been adopted by Alcino and Karen really rests on whether the Children's Status Act was designed to be retrospective. Professor Tager believes it was.

She says:

> Laws are not usually retrospective, unless they operate for the benefit of the individual. A child who was born as a result of artificial insemination before the Act came into operation would be illegitimate if the law did not operate retrospectively. Surely, therefore, it is arguable that the law must be altered to be of benefit to that child and operate retrospectively. This leads me to the conclusion that children born to a married woman who has been artificially inseminated with her husband's consent even before the Act came into operation are covered by this law.

And she added:

> I would not have agreed to the registration of these triplets in the name of Karen, the daughter. Mrs Anthony gave birth to the children and therefore she would be the mother. There is a strong argument for saying that the triplets are Mrs Anthony's legitimate children.
>
> Certainly our new Children's Status Act in South Africa puts it beyond doubt that if there was another case like the Anthony one today, the surrogate mother's child would be the legitimate offspring of her marriage.

In a paper published in 1988, Susan Bedil, lecturer in law at the Witwatersrand University, also says that the new law means that the triplets are the legitimate children of the woman who received artificial insemination, Pat Anthony.

By applying this interpretation to the Anthony case, it follows that these triplets are the 'brothers' and 'sister' of their 'biological' mother, Karen Ferreira-Jorge.

The fact that there was an agreement between the parties concerned that the grandmother would hand the children over to her daughter and the father, and that the children were allowed to be registered in the name of their biological parents, does not in law make the biological parents the lawful parents.

Her paper adds: 'I believe adoption is the only way that the triplets concerned may become the children of the Ferreira-Jorges.'

Susan Bedil, like Professor Tager, believes that the Children's Status Act was drawn up to operate retrospectively so that the fact that it was enacted a fortnight after the birth of the triplets is an irrelevance.

However Rika Pretorius, of the University of South Africa law faculty, and also an expert on surrogacy, wrote a letter to the South African attorneys' journal, *De Rebus*, earlier in 1988 insisting that the Ferreira-Jorge triplets were legally the babies of Karen and Alcino because they had been born before the Act became law.

'Had the Ferreira-Jorge triplets been born two weeks later they would have been the legitimate children of Mr and Mrs Anthony and brothers and sister of their biological parents.'

Rika Pretorius pointed out that the Act itself was a positive step towards legislation to legitimize the children born as a result of artificial insemination with donor sperm in South Africa. Previously these children would have been illegitimate.

But she warned:

> This Act has complicated contractual surrogacy arrangements in South Africa considerably. It terminates the

rights, obligations and duties of the semen and ova donors – the genetic parents – towards the child.

A donor will no longer be able to claim parental rights to the child, and the children will not be able to claim maintenance from a donor. This affects cases of full surrogacy where the genetic material of the commissioning couple is fertilized in a test tube and the surrogate mother merely carries the child to term. As in the Ferreira-Jorge case.

Such children are now considered to be the legitimate children of surrogate mothers and their husbands, provided their husbands consent to the artificial insemination. He does not even have to put that consent in writing.

Today test-tube baby-making is being practised in 25 countries, including most of Western Europe, Columbia, Chile, the People's Republic of China, East Germany, Denmark, Japan and Singapore. Each one of these nations is grappling to produce safeguards which will protect the children of such medical experimentation. But it will only be when these 'Brave New World' offspring are grown up that the real consequences of *in-vitro* fertilization and the use of surrogate mothers will be known. Then these young people – like David, Jose and Paula – will be able to speak for themselves about their own extraordinary creation.